Interventions to Promote Physical Activity and Healthy Ageing

Interventions to Promote Physical Activity and Healthy Ageing

Guest Editors
Andy Pringle
Nicola Kime

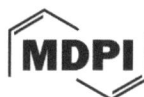

Basel • Beijing • Wuhan • Barcelona • Belgrade • Novi Sad • Cluj • Manchester

Guest Editors

Andy Pringle
Clinical Exercise and
Rehabilitation Research Centre
University of Derby
Derby
United Kingdom

Nicola Kime
Academic Unit for Ageing
and Stroke Research
Bradford Institute for
Health Research
Bradford
United Kingdom

Editorial Office
MDPI AG
Grosspeteranlage 5
4052 Basel, Switzerland

This is a reprint of the Special Issue, published open access by the journal *International Journal of Environmental Research and Public Health* (ISSN 1660-4601), freely accessible at: www.mdpi.com/journal/ijerph/special_issues/aging_physical_intervention.

For citation purposes, cite each article independently as indicated on the article page online and using the guide below:

Lastname, A.A.; Lastname, B.B. Article Title. *Journal Name* **Year**, *Volume Number*, Page Range.

ISBN 978-3-7258-2880-7 (Hbk)
ISBN 978-3-7258-2879-1 (PDF)
https://doi.org/10.3390/books978-3-7258-2879-1

Cover image courtesy of Andy Pringle

© 2025 by the authors. Articles in this book are Open Access and distributed under the Creative Commons Attribution (CC BY) license. The book as a whole is distributed by MDPI under the terms and conditions of the Creative Commons Attribution-NonCommercial-NoDerivs (CC BY-NC-ND) license (https://creativecommons.org/licenses/by-nc-nd/4.0/).

Contents

About the Editors vii

Preface ix

Andy Pringle and Nicky Kime
Interventions to Promote Physical Activity and Healthy Ageing: An Editorial
Reprinted from: *Int. J. Environ. Res. Public Health* **2024**, *21*, 1225,
https://doi.org/10.3390/ijerph21091225 1

Nichola M. Davis, Andy Pringle, Anthony D. Kay, Anthony J. Blazevich, Danielle Teskey and Mark A. Faghy et al.
Feasibility, Psychosocial Effects, Influence, and Perception of Elastic Band Resistance Balance Training in Older Adults
Reprinted from: *Int. J. Environ. Res. Public Health* **2022**, *19*, 10907,
https://doi.org/10.3390/ijerph191710907 4

Marcelo de Maio Nascimento, Élvio Rúbio Gouveia, Adilson Marques, Bruna R. Gouveia, Priscila Marconcin and Cíntia França et al.
The Role of Physical Function in the Association between Physical Activity and Gait Speed in Older Adults: A Mediation Analysis
Reprinted from: *Int. J. Environ. Res. Public Health* **2022**, *19*, 12581,
https://doi.org/10.3390/ijerph191912581 24

Cheng-En Wu, Kai Way Li, Fan Chia and Wei-Yang Huang
Interventions to Improve Physical Capability of Older Adults with Mild Disabilities: A Case Study
Reprinted from: *Int. J. Environ. Res. Public Health* **2022**, *19*, 2651,
https://doi.org/10.3390/ijerph19052651 39

Alba Niño, José Gerardo Villa-Vicente and Pilar S. Collado
Functional Capacity of Tai Chi-Practicing Elderly People
Reprinted from: *Int. J. Environ. Res. Public Health* **2022**, *19*, 2178,
https://doi.org/10.3390/ijerph19042178 50

Angela Devereux-Fitzgerald, Rachael Powell and David P. French
The Acceptability of Physical Activity to Older Adults Living in Lower Socioeconomic Status Areas: A Multi-Perspective Study
Reprinted from: *Int. J. Environ. Res. Public Health* **2021**, *18*, 11784,
https://doi.org/10.3390/ijerph182211784 61

Conor Cunningham and Roger O'Sullivan
Healthcare Professionals Promotion of Physical Activity with Older Adults: A Survey of Knowledge and Routine Practice
Reprinted from: *Int. J. Environ. Res. Public Health* **2021**, *18*, 6064,
https://doi.org/10.3390/ijerph18116064 74

Conor Cunningham and Roger O'Sullivan
Healthcare Professionals' Application and Integration of Physical Activity in Routine Practice with Older Adults: A Qualitative Study
Reprinted from: *Int. J. Environ. Res. Public Health* **2021**, *18*, 11222,
https://doi.org/10.3390/ijerph182111222 87

Mark Cortnage and Andy Pringle
Onset of Weight Gain and Health Concerns for Men: Findings from the TAP Programme
Reprinted from: *Int. J. Environ. Res. Public Health* **2022**, *19*, 579,
https://doi.org/10.3390/ijerph19010579 . . . . **106**

J. Yoon Irons, Alison Williams, Jo Holland and Julie Jones
An Exploration of People Living with Parkinson's Experience of Cardio-Drumming; Parkinson's Beats: A Qualitative Phenomenological Study
Reprinted from: *Int. J. Environ. Res. Public Health* **2024**, *21*, 514,
https://doi.org/10.3390/ijerph21040514 . . . . **121**

Christopher Russell
"We Can Do This!": The Role of Physical Activity in What Comes Next for Dementia
Reprinted from: *Int. J. Environ. Res. Public Health* **2023**, *20*, 6503,
https://doi.org/10.3390/ijerph20156503 . . . . **133**

About the Editors

Andy Pringle

Andy Pringle is a Professor of Physical Activity and Health Intervention and the Research Centre Lead for the Clinical Exercise and Rehabilitation Research Centre and the School of Sport and Exercise Sciences at the University of Derby. Andy's research investigates the impact and implementation of physical activity interventions. He has published over 100 peer-reviewed articles and book chapters. Andy is also a Visiting Professor at the University of Leeds, a Fellow of the Royal Society of Public Health, and a NICE Guidelines Implementation Expert. He was involved in the 2019 UK Chief Medical Officers' (CMO) Physical Activity Guidelines and was a member of the UK Expert Committee for Communications that informs the four UK CMOs on communication priorities for physical activity. He worked on the NICE Guidelines for Exercise Referral 2014 and Walking and Cycling (Exceptional Update, 2018). In 2023, Andy was appointed a 'Topic Expert' on the 'Prioritization' of the NICE Physical Activity Guidance. He is also a member of the Sport England National Evaluation Learning Partner Expert Reference Group, 2022. By 2024, Andy had supervised 10 PhD students to successful completion and performed 16 postgraduate research student examinations. He has a PhD investigating the impact and implementation of community physical activity interventions and an M.Sc. in Health Promotion and Public Health. He is also trained in intervention mapping techniques and has extensive experience evaluating community physical activity and health interventions at the local and national level for a range of organisations.

Nicola Kime

Dr Nicky Kime is a Senior Research Fellow working on the NIHR RfPB, a qualitative exploration of older women and healthcare practitioner experiences to guide improvements in osteoporosis care, and the NIHR HS&DR, developing the evidence and associated service model to support older people living with frailty to manage their pain and to reduce its impact on their lives: a mixed-method, co-design study. Nicky has extensive experience with leading and managing applied research and consultancy projects for a range of organisations, predominantly in the NHS but also including charities, local government departments, and schools. Prior to joining the Academic Unit for Ageing and Stroke Research, Nicky's work focused on long-term conditions, predominantly the care of children, young people, and adults with type 1; service improvement; physical activity and behaviour change; and the education and training of healthcare professionals. Nicky's main areas of expertise are qualitative methodology and methods and evaluation research. Nicky has an MSc in Health Promotion/Public Health and a PhD in Children's Eating Behaviours and Intergenerational Influences.

Preface

The Healthy Ageing Challenge aims for people to enjoy at least five extra healthy independent years of life by 2035 while narrowing the gap between the experiences of the richest and poorest. Regular physical activity is important for healthy ageing, not only for maintaining health in midlife but also for maintaining health, independence, and quality of life as people become older. Global physical activity guidelines highlight the benefits and importance of helping adults to adopt and maintain regular physical activity participation throughout the course of life and not only in later life, and interventions and activities that support this aspiration are so important. As experienced researchers, Professor Andy Pringle and Dr Nicky Kime's text, Interventions to Promote Physical Activity and Healthy Ageing, features contributions reporting the impact and implementation of physical activity interventions for adults and older adults, as well as the experiences of performing research and evaluation in this context in a diverse range of projects. The text provides important learning for practice and research in physical activity and public health. As such, it will be of interest to colleagues working in the design, implementation, and evaluation/research of physical activity interventions for adults and older adults.

Andy Pringle and Nicola Kime
Guest Editors

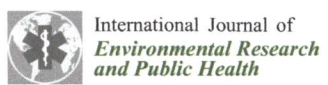

Editorial

Interventions to Promote Physical Activity and Healthy Ageing: An Editorial

Andy Pringle [1,*] and Nicky Kime [2]

1. Clinical Exercise and Rehabilitation Research Centre, School of Sport and Exercise Science, University of Derby, Kedleston Road, Derby DE22 1GB, UK
2. Bradford Institute for Health Research, Temple Bank House, Bradford Royal Infirmary, Bradford BD9 6RJ, UK
* Correspondence: a.pringle@derby.ac.uk

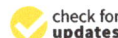

Citation: Pringle, A.; Kime, N. Interventions to Promote Physical Activity and Healthy Ageing: An Editorial. *Int. J. Environ. Res. Public Health* **2024**, *21*, 1225. https://doi.org/10.3390/ijerph21091225

Received: 6 September 2024
Accepted: 14 September 2024
Published: 18 September 2024

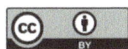

Copyright: © 2024 by the authors. Licensee MDPI, Basel, Switzerland. This article is an open access article distributed under the terms and conditions of the Creative Commons Attribution (CC BY) license (https://creativecommons.org/licenses/by/4.0/).

The Healthy Ageing Challenge aims for people to enjoy at least five extra healthy, independent years of life by 2035, while narrowing the gap between the experiences of the richest and poorest. Regular physical activity is important for healthy ageing, not only for maintaining health in midlife but also for maintaining health, independence and quality of life as people become older. Physical activity guidelines highlight the benefits and the importance of helping adults to adopt and maintain regular physical activity participation throughout the life course and not only in later life, and interventions and activities that support this aspiration are so important. We are delighted that this Special Issue features contributions that report both the impact and implementation of physical activity interventions for adults and older adults, as well as a range of studies on this topic [1]. Research highlights the importance of physical activity in maintaining functionality and retaining independence, in order that people can do all the things they want and need to do in their daily life [2,3]. One of the key features of the most recent UK physical activity guidelines is a greater emphasis being placed on activities that promote strength and balance [3]. Several of the papers in this Special Issue focus on this important topic, along with physical functioning [Contributions 1–4]. With those thoughts in mind, Davis and colleagues investigate the feasibility, psychosocial effects, influence, and perception of elastic band resistance balance training in older adults [Contribution 1]. Their pilot work also investigates the preferences, likes, and dislikes of older adults regarding the exercises. Understanding what works well and what works less well, and the reasons for this is important, as reiterated by Davis and several other studies in this collection. Indeed, holding dialogue with participants about their physical activity needs, preferences, likes, and dislikes is important in shaping the design and delivery of interventions. Devereux and colleagues remind us that some older adults in lower socioeconomic status (SES) areas are among the least active of all adult groups but are often absent from physical activity research. It is valuable that their study aimed to elicit important perspectives on the acceptability of physical activity from both the perspectives of older adults and physical activity providers [Contribution 5].

When we consider the providers of advice on physical activity, healthcare professionals (HCPs) are important agents for promoting physical activity to adults and older adults [3,4]. Cunningham and O'Sullivan explored HCPs' knowledge, decision making, and routine practice of physical activity promotion with older adults [Contributions 6–7]. Less than a third of respondents had a clear plan on how to initiate discussions about physical activity in routine practice with older adults [Contribution 6]. Understanding the barriers that HCPs face when promoting physical activity is important. Research has investigated the role of doctors in promoting physical activity, including the barriers and facilitators they face in doing so [4]. Given the key role that HCPs play and, in some instances, their lack of preparedness for promoting a physically active lifestyle, insights are important in shaping activities which help support HCPs preparations in helping people to adopt physical activity [Contribution 6–7]. Although HCPs have been identified as key conduits for promoting physical activity [3,4], there are other individuals and agencies that also have a role to play. The importance of local community agencies in helping people start and keep physically active has long been identified [5]. Health interventions delivered through community-based agencies, foundations, and charities are an important part of the public health landscape, especially given a declining range of public services from some statutory bodies. One key feature of the offer made by community providers is connecting to people around their interests, including their leisure preferences. With this in mind, Cortnage's study illustrates how to connect men to health improvement programmes through the power of football [Contribution 8]. Thinking about people's active recreation preferences, it was, also, great to receive Iron's 'Parkinson Beats' study, exploring people with Parkinson's experience of cardio-drumming [Contribution 9]. In this spirit, Russell's review, '"We Can Do This!": The Role of Physical Activity in What Comes Next for Dementia', focuses upon life with dementia and the role that physical activity can play within it [Contribution 10]. Indeed, several of our studies focus on adults with long-term conditions, including Wu's case study, which explores interventions to improve the physical capability of older adults with mild disabilities [Contribution 3]. Finally, all our contributions to this Special Issue [1] provide valuable insights on undertaking research and evaluation within this context and provide learning to inform future investigations on this topic. This Special Issue brings together an eclectic mix of studies, including contributions from an international authorship [Contributions 2–4], which add to the insights provided in this body of work.

Nicky and I are pleased that early career researchers have also taken up the call to submit their work. Helping researchers to publish is something that we are passionate about. In this respect, we are grateful for the support our early career researchers received from more experienced colleagues, as well as the support offered by the editorial team at *IJERPH*. We are also grateful to every author who submitted to our call for papers [24 papers in total], especially to the authors whose papers were eventually included in other *IJERPH* Special Issues. We are grateful to our independent peer reviewers who provided feedback on the submissions, along with the thousands of readers who have already accessed this Special Issue. Finally, we thank all the people and professionals who took part in and supported the research featured in this Special Issue, which helped grow our understanding and knowledge of this important area of work.

We hope to follow this collection of works with a second edition, but for now, Nicky and I hope you enjoy reading this Special Issue.

Author Contributions: Conceptualization, A.P. and N.K.; methodology, A.P. and N.K.; validation, A.P., and N.K.; formal analysis, A.P. and N.K.; investigation, A.P. and N.K.; resources, A.P. and N.K.; writing—original draft preparation, A.P. and N.K.; writing—review and editing, A.P. and N.K.; visualization, A.P. and N.K.; project administration, A.P. and N.K.; funding acquisition, A.P. and N.K. All authors have read and agreed to the published version of the manuscript.

Conflicts of Interest: Where the editors are also the authors of any articles in this Special Issue, these submissions have been subjected to independent internal and external peer-review processes and protocols for this journal.

List of Contributions

1. Davis, N.M.; Pringle, A.; Kay, A.D.; Blazevich, A.J.; Teskey, D.; Faghy, M.A.; Mina, M.A. Feasibility, Psychosocial Effects, Influence, and Perception of Elastic Band Resistance Balance Training in Older Adults. *Int. J. Environ. Res. Public Health* **2022**, *19*, 10907. https://doi.org/10.3390/ijerph191710907.
2. Nascimento, M.d.M.; Gouveia, É.R.; Marques, A.; Gouveia, B.R.; Marconcin, P.; França, C.; Ihle, A. The Role of Physical Function in the Association between Physical Activity and Gait Speed in Older Adults: A Mediation Analysis. *Int. J. Environ. Res. Public Health* **2022**, *19*, 12581. https://doi.org/10.3390/ijerph191912581.
3. Wu, C.-E.; Li, K.W.; Chia, F.; Huang, W.-Y. Interventions to Improve Physical Capability of Older Adults with Mild Disabilities: A Case Study. *Int. J. Environ. Res. Public Health* **2022**, *19*, 2651. https://doi.org/10.3390/ijerph19052651

4. Niño, A.; Villa-Vicente, J.G.; S. Collado, P. Functional Capacity of Tai Chi-Practicing Elderly People. *Int. J. Environ. Res. Public Health* **2022**, *19*, 2178. https://doi.org/10.3390/ijerph19042178
5. Devereux-Fitzgerald, A.; Powell, R.; French, D.P. The Acceptability of Physical Activity to Older Adults Living in Lower Socioeconomic Status Areas: A Multi-Perspective Study. *Int. J. Environ. Res. Public Health* **2021**, *18*, 11784. https://doi.org/10.3390/ijerph182211784
6. Cunningham, C.; O'Sullivan, R. Healthcare Professionals Promotion of Physical Activity with Older Adults: A Survey of Knowledge and Routine Practice. *Int. J. Environ. Res. Public Health* **2021**, *18*, 6064. https://doi.org/10.3390/ijerph18116064
7. Cunningham, C.; O'Sullivan, R. Healthcare Professionals' Application and Integration of Physical Activity in Routine Practice with Older Adults: A Qualitative Study. *Int. J. Environ. Res. Public Health* **2021**, *18*, 11222. https://doi.org/10.3390/ijerph182111222
8. Cortnage, M.; Pringle, A. Onset of Weight Gain and Health Concerns for Men: Findings from the TAP Programme. *Int. J. Environ. Res. Public Health* **2022**, *19*, 579. https://doi.org/10.3390/ijerph19010579
9. Irons, J.Y.; Williams, A.; Holland, J.; Jones, J. An Exploration of People Living with Parkinson's Experience of Cardio-Drumming; Parkinson's Beats: A Qualitative Phenomenological Study. *Int. J. Environ. Res. Public Health* **2024**, *21*, 514. https://doi.org/10.3390/ijerph21040514
10. Russell, C. "We Can Do This!": The Role of Physical Activity in What Comes Next for Dementia. *Int. J. Environ. Res. Public Health* **2023**, *20*, 6503. https://doi.org/10.3390/ijerph20156503

References

1. Interventions to Promote Physical Activity and Healthy Ageing: Special Issue. *Int. J. Environ. Res. Public Health* (ISSN 1660-4601). Available online: https://www.mdpi.com/journal/ijerph/special_issues/aging_physical_intervention (accessed on 10 September 2024).
2. Skelton, D.A.; Copeland, R.J.; Tew, G.A.; Mavroeidi, A.; Cleather, D.J.; Stathi, A.; Greig, C.A.; Tully, M.A. Expert Working Group Working Paper UK Physical Activity Guidelines: Older Adults Working Group. Review and Recommendations for Older Adults (Aged 65+ Years). Available online: https://www.bristol.ac.uk/media-library/sites/sps/documents/cmo/older-adults-technical-report.pdf (accessed on 10 September 2024).
3. Department of Health and Social Care. Physical Activity Guidelines: UK Chief Medical Officers' Report. A Report from the Chief Medical Officers in the UK on the Amount and Type of Physical Activity People Should Be Doing to Improve Their Health. London, 2018. Available online: https://www.gov.uk/government/publications/physical-activity-guidelines-uk-chief-medical-officers-report (accessed on 10 September 2024).
4. Vishnubala, D.; Iqbal, A.; Marino, K.; Whatmough, S.; Barker, R.; Salman, D.; Bazira, P.; Finn, G.; Pringle, A.; Nykjaer, C. UK Doctors Delivering Physical Activity Advice: What Are the Challenges and Possible Solutions? A Qualitative Study. *Int. J. Environ. Res. Public Health* **2022**, *19*, 12030. [CrossRef] [PubMed]
5. Goodman, C.; Davies, S.; Tai, S.S.; Dinan, S.; Iliffe, S. Promoting older peoples' participation in activity, whose responsibility? A case study of the response of health, local government and voluntary organizations. *J. Interprof. Care* **2007**, *21*, 515–528. [CrossRef] [PubMed]

Disclaimer/Publisher's Note: The statements, opinions and data contained in all publications are solely those of the individual author(s) and contributor(s) and not of MDPI and/or the editor(s). MDPI and/or the editor(s) disclaim responsibility for any injury to people or property resulting from any ideas, methods, instructions or products referred to in the content.

Article

Feasibility, Psychosocial Effects, Influence, and Perception of Elastic Band Resistance Balance Training in Older Adults

Nichola M. Davis [1,*], Andy Pringle [1], Anthony D. Kay [2], Anthony J. Blazevich [3], Danielle Teskey [1], Mark A. Faghy [1] and Minas A. Mina [1]

1 Department of Sport, Outdoor and Exercise Science, School of Human Sciences & Human Sciences Research Centre, University of Derby, Kedleston Road, Derby DE22 1GB, UK
2 Centre for Physical Activity & Life Sciences, University of Northampton, Northampton NN2 7AL, UK
3 Centre for Human Performance, School of Medical & Health Sciences, Edith Cowan University, Joondalup, WA 6027, Australia
* Correspondence: n.davis@derby.ac.uk

Abstract: This study utilised feedback from older adults during balance-challenging, elastic band resistance exercises to design a physical activity (PA) intervention. Methods: Twenty-three active participants, aged 51–81 years, volunteered to perform a mini balance evaluation test and falls efficacy scale, and completed a daily living questionnaire. Following a 10 min warm-up, participants performed eight pre-selected exercises (1 × set, 8–12 repetitions) using elastic bands placed over the hip or chest regions in a randomised, counterbalanced order with 15 min seated rests between interventions. Heart rate (HR) and rate of perceived exertion (RPE) were measured throughout. Participant interview responses were used to qualify the experiences and opinions of the interventions including likes, dislikes, comfort, and exercise difficulty. Results: Similar significant ($p < 0.01$) increases in HR (pre- = 83–85 bpm, mid- = 85–88 bpm, post-intervention = 88–89 bpm; 5–6%) and RPE (pre- = 8–9, mid- = 10, post-intervention = 10–11) were detected during the PA interventions (hip and chest regions). Interview data revealed that participants thought the PA interventions challenged balance, that the exercises would be beneficial for balance, and that the exercises were suitable for themselves and others. Participants reported a positive experience when using the PA interventions with an elastic band placed at the hip or chest and would perform the exercises again, preferably in a group, and that individual preference and comfort would determine the placement of the elastic band at either the hip or chest. Conclusion: These positive outcomes confirm the feasibility of a resistance band balance program and will inform intervention design and delivery in future studies.

Keywords: postural control; elderly; resistance bands; falls prevention; physical activity

1. Introduction

Fall-related accidents are a key national UK public health priority with fragility fractures estimated an annual cost of GBP 4.4 billion [1]. Furthermore, the impact of fall-related accidents may lead to injury, pain, fear of falling, loss of independence and confidence, mobility limitations, and mortality [2]. Age-related declines in both the sensory (vision, vestibular, and proprioception) and neuromuscular (strength, power, range of motion) systems negatively affect postural stability, which is an important factor for older adults to perform usual activities of daily life such as walking, turning, moving, and functioning independently [3]. Impaired balance control increases the risk of falls in older adults due to the difficulty in controlling balance recovery reactions, e.g., swaying around the ankles or hips, and taking steps beyond the base of support [4,5]. Therefore, developing physical activity (PA) interventions to improve/maintain postural control is important not only for overall health and psychological benefits but also for daily functioning and independence [6]. Understanding the key facilitators and barriers that older adults may face when adopting and maintaining PA is crucial when developing feasible, accessible, appropriate, affordable, and enjoyable interventions [7], including those centred on fall prevention.

The determinants for participation in PA by older adults have been identified in the development of the social ecological model (SEM) [7], which highlights enjoyment, sociable, affordable, accessible, and flexible as important aspects of a PA program for older adults [7]. Additionally, the self-determination theory of human motivation supports the concept of psychological needs, autonomy competence, and enjoyment as influences on behavioural motivation for participation in PA [8,9]. These findings emphasise the importance of obtaining feedback on newly designed PA interventions to ensure that they meet the needs of older adults. Many PA interventions examine task-specific reactive balance, which is recommended as an optimal intervention for improving reactive balance in older adults [5,10]. Perturbation-based balance training aims to incorporate repeated postural perturbations to evoke instantaneous rapid balance reactions to reduce falls in older adults [11–13] with the potential of producing quicker adaptations to improve balance compared to conventional balance training [13]. Furthermore, perturbation-based balance training is an approach used in fall prevention with improved balance, confidence [14], resilience, and balance reactive control to respond to real-life circumstances such as trips that occur in daily life [15]. Such interventions are often performed in clinical settings and are not always accessible to all older adults as part of a regular exercise regime.

Muscular strength is another important factor for maintaining balance, which is recommended in PA guidelines for older adults [16]. Strength reductions in ageing have been associated with muscle changes, leading to increased risk of falls and difficulty in performing daily tasks such as climbing stairs, rising from a chair, and household chores. The importance of muscular strength highlights the need to include strengthening exercises in PA interventions for older adults, which can be achieved using elastic band resistance [17]. Studies documenting the use of elastic band resistance versus conventional resistance training using weight machines have shown similar improvements in strength [18], isometric force [19], peripheral muscle force [17], functional exercise capacity [20], and improvements in health-related quality of life in older adults [19]. Elastic band resistance is a useful, cost-effective, and safe intervention in the rehabilitation of balance impairments in older adults [21]. When used in a full-body training program, elastic band resistance has been shown to improve postural control in older adults [22,23], and in targeted lower limb strengthening training has been shown to influence balance, gait function, flexibility, and fall efficacy [24]. However, the importance of involving and engaging older adults in the development of interventions that meet their needs and preferences is a critical factor for a successful PA intervention [7,25]. Furthermore, to our knowledge, the use of elastic band resistance to challenge balance using this methodology within the individual's base of support (similar to that of perturbation-based balance training) has not been previously examined. Given the above, this study aimed to develop a novel PA intervention using elastic band resistance training to challenge balance and utilise the perspectives of older adults to shape an accessible, appropriate, and acceptable intervention for older adults to meet their needs.

2. Materials and Methods

2.1. Participants

Twenty-three healthy and moderately physically active older adults (66.5 ± 8.3 years) (Table 1) were recruited through existing physical activity networks in the Derbyshire community to participate in the study after completing written, informed consent and a PA health screening questionnaire. Inclusion criteria included individuals (1) over 50 years of age, (2) having the ability to walk without a walking aid, (3) achieving an activity level score of >600 MET-min per week according to the International PA Readiness Questionnaire (IPAQ), and (4) achieving a score of >23 in the Mini-Mental State Examination (MMSE). Exclusion criteria included participants with (1) unstable cardiovascular conditions, (2) acute respiratory disease, (3) Parkinson's disease, (4) Huntington's disease, (5) acute stroke,

(6) lower limb paresis, or (7) uncontrolled diabetes mellitus. Fall history was recorded for the previous 6 months with no participants reporting a fall. A falls efficacy scale, International Activity of Daily Living Questionnaire, and a mini balance evaluation test were completed prior to taking part in the PA intervention. This study was conducted as part of a feasibility trial designed to evaluate the intervention design of a novel PA intervention using elastic band resistance. Attendance of a single experimental trial at the University of Derby (UK) was required. A mixed-methods design was implemented using qualitative and quantitative data to help evaluate and understand the feasibility of the PA interventions. Ethical approval was granted by the Human Science Research Ethics Committee at the University of Derby (ID: ETH2021/4503) in July 2021. The study was clinically registered (ClinicalTrials.gov ID: NCT04932408).

Table 1. Descriptive characteristics of participant demographics.

Demographic Characteristics	All Participants (n = 23)
Age (years)	66.5 ± 8 (51–81 years)
Body mass (kg)	83 ± 15
Height (cm)	165 ± 12
IPAQ	High
MMSE	29 ± 1
IADL	8 ± 1
FES-I	9 ± 4
Mini BESTest	26 ± 3

Notes: values presented as mean ± standard deviation. IPAQ: international physical activity questionnaire, FES-I: falls efficacy scale, IADL: International Activity of Daily Living questionnaire, MMSE: mini mental state examination, Mini BESTest: mini balance evaluation test.

2.2. Study Design

A randomised, counterbalanced design was implemented to compare two PA interventions using elastic bands placed at the hip and the chest region on the same day in a single session. Each participant performed the intervention between 10:00 a.m. and 2:00 p.m. to control for time-of-day effects on balance performance, including accumulation of general tiredness and general muscle fatigue. Randomisation was performed for both the order of the PA interventions (either the hip or chest placement first) and the order in which the exercises were performed. Following a 10 min supervised warm-up, all participants performed 8 pre-selected exercises for 1 × 12 repetitions (performed for 30 min on average) (Figure 1) with the elastic band placed at either the hip or chest with a 15 min seated rest before completing the second intervention with the elastic band placed at either the hip or chest (Figures 1 and 2). Heart rate (HR) and rate of perceived exertion (RPE) were recorded before, during (6th repetition), and after each exercise. Refinement of the methods during the piloting phases of the study can be found in Supplementary File S1. Following the PA interventions, participants were invited to take part in a semi-structured interview with a digital voice recorder and written notes taken during the interview.

Hip region   Chest region

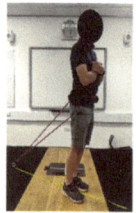 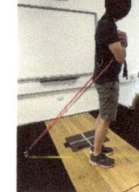

1. **Forward step:** Step forward with both feet with concentric hold for 4 seconds.

Figure 1. *Cont.*

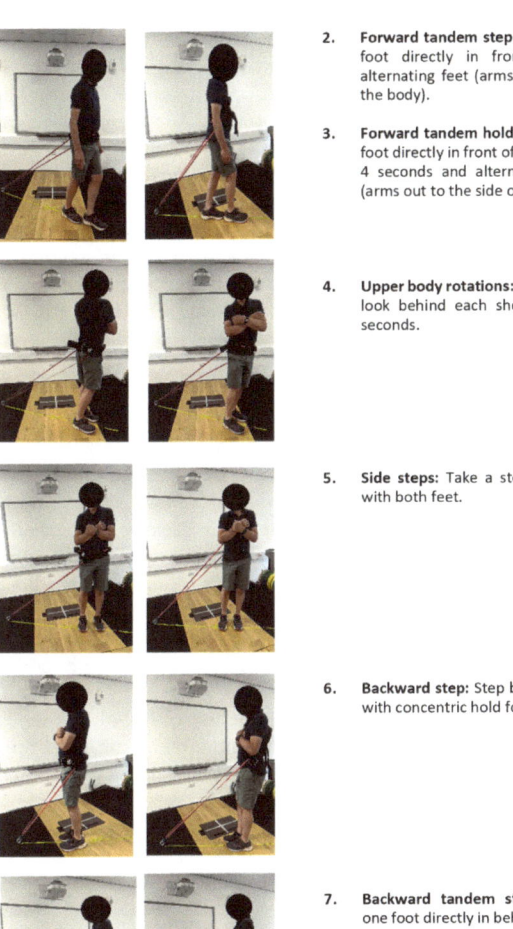

2. **Forward tandem step:** Placement of one foot directly in front of the other, alternating feet (arms out to the side of the body).

3. **Forward tandem hold:** Placement of one foot directly in front of the other, hold for 4 seconds and alternate to other foot (arms out to the side of the body).

4. **Upper body rotations:** Cross arms, turn to look behind each shoulder, hold for 4 seconds.

5. **Side steps:** Take a step out to the side with both feet.

6. **Backward step:** Step back with both feet with concentric hold for 4 seconds.

7. **Backward tandem step:** Placement of one foot directly in behind the other (heel to toe), alternating feet (arms out to the side of the body).

8. **Backward tandem hold:** Placement of one foot directly in behind the other, hold for 4 seconds and alternate to other foot (arms out to the side of the body).

Figure 1. Examples of the elastic band resistance exercises in each PA intervention (hip and chest regions).

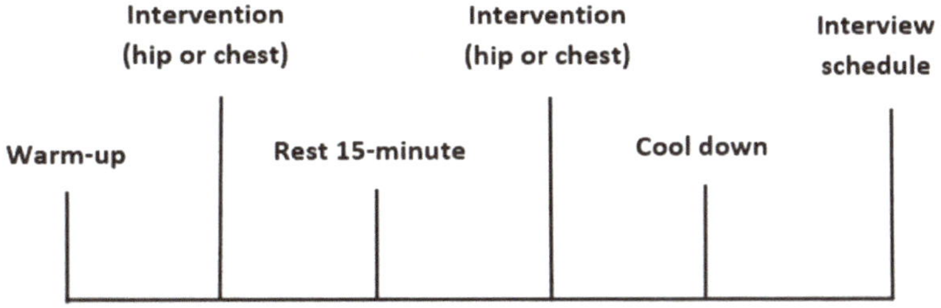

Figure 2. Study design timeline of the intervention protocol.

2.3. Interviews with Participants

Interviews took place between July and October 2021 with data collected using semi-structured interviews lasting approximately 30 min. The aim of the interviews was to identify the determinants, opinions, and perceptions of the PA intervention to shape subsequent intervention design. This included scaling questions on difficulty, comfort, and enjoyment of the exercise selection and further questions related to personal preferences on the exercise selection, comfort, difficulty, modality, suitability, perceived benefits, safety, environmental factors, and the exercise equipment to determine the feasibility of the PA intervention. The interview schedule was developed through prior knowledge of creating PA interventions [7], and this type of approach has been used previously in PA research to provide in-depth and insightful accounts with professionals [26] and older adult participants [27,28]. The interview schedule is available upon request from the corresponding author.

2.4. Data Analysis

Analyses were performed using SPSS (version 26, IBM Corporation, Armonk, NY, USA) with all data reported as mean (M) ± standard deviation (SD). Normal distribution was assessed using the Shapiro–Wilk test; no significant difference ($p > 0.05$) was detected in any variable, indicating that all data sets were normally distributed. Separate two-way repeated measures ANOVAs (2×3) were used to determine between (condition $\times$ 2) and within (time $\times$ 3) effects on HR and RPE measures. Post hoc t-tests were performed to determine the location of any significant differences.

Participant interviews were recorded and manually transcribed verbatim by the lead researcher; all names were altered to a pseudonym code for use in the results to ensure anonymity. Following reading of the transcripts to saturation, template analysis was performed, which encourages the use of initial themes. The priori themes included the exercise band placement, environmental factors, and the exercise preferences. This type of analysis uses a hierarchical coding and offers researchers a high degree of structure; however, this approach also allows for flexibility of the structure, which was required for the analysis in this study [29,30]. Template analysis was used to guide a thematic analysis process [31]: (1) coding to identify interesting features of the data; (2) grouping into sub-themes to provide a systematic framework, and (3) a visual map developed by hand to show the themes and their relationships. Three main themes were defined: (1) perceptions on exercise selection, (2) opinions on the exercise equipment/elastic band placement location, and (3) participant views on the environment factors. These finalised themes were used to guide the analysis and organise the qualitative findings.

3. Results

3.1. Demographics and Participant Profile

Tables 1 and 2 show the demographics of the interviewed participants.

Table 2. Demographic profile of the participants.

Participant	Gender	Ethnicity	Age Group (Years)
1	M	White British	75–84
2	F	British	75–84
3	F	British	65–74
4	F	White British	75–84
5	M	British	65–74
6	F	White British	50–54
7	F	White British	65–74
8	F	White British	65–74
9	F	White British	65–74
10	F	White British	55–64

Table 2. Cont.

Participant	Gender	Ethnicity	Age Group (Years)
11	F	White British	55–64
12	M	African	55–64
13	F	White British	65–74
14	F	White British	65–74
15	F	White British	65–74
16	M	White British	55–64
17	F	White British	75–84
18	M	White British	50–54
19	M	White British	75–84
20	M	White British	55–64
21	M	White British	50–54
22	M	White British	65–74
23	M	White British	65–74

Notes: gender M = male, F = female.

3.2. Interviews with Participants

Participant reports were organised using themes and sub-themes (see details below). Following analysis, priori themes were merged into three final themes based on the emerging data set: (1) perceptions of the exercise selection, (2) opinions of the exercise equipment, and (3) insights into the preferred environment (Figure 3). Multiple data sets describe the key findings of the participant feedback on the PA intervention through the interview schedules performed and the perceived intensity of the PA intervention recorded by HR and RPE measures.

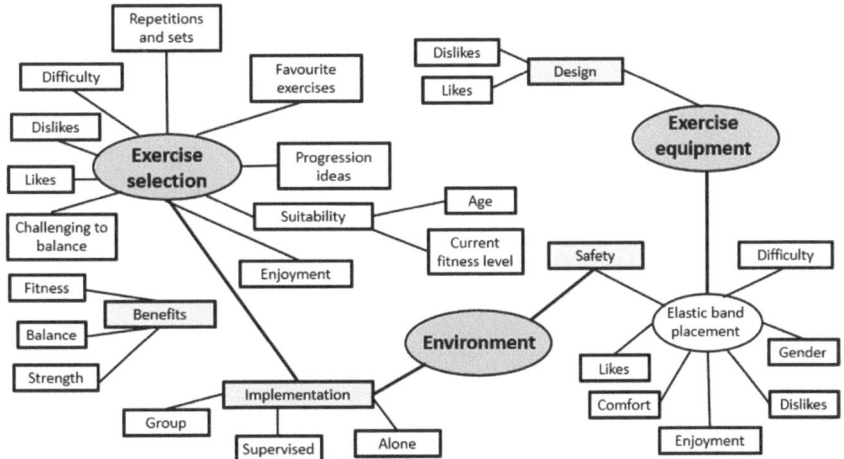

Figure 3. Figure to illustrate the key themes and the interconnectivity of the themes and sub-themes.

3.3. Participants' Perceptions of the Exercise Selection

3.3.1. The PA Intervention and Balance

Participants reported their perceptions on the exercises that challenged balance whilst performing them using an elastic resistance band. This is illustrated by the following quotes:

- "The tandem steps, it seemed to me that you only have to be a fraction out and the bands sort of accentuate it and pull you off balance further". (P19)
- "I just felt a bit out of sync, you know, wobbly again. That's when I'm putting my foot back like that (tandem stance) I find them a bit wobbly. It does challenge your balance, but it's nice. It's all right". (P14)

- "Definitely everything involving going backwards. Especially if you need to do it under pressure, you know because you're doing it with band you are you are doing it against something rather than just doing it without as just walking does". (P4)

Participants reported some of the exercises did not challenge their balance as such:

- "Upper body rotations did not challenge my balance, not at all. And the side steps not at all. I seem to function well stepping sideways". (P9)
- "I wouldn't have said the walking one challenged the balance too much (forward and backward steps). But I thought that was quite a good exercise because it felt like to me like walking uphill and it's got to be got to be good for you. That might be the most cardio-intensive one you know". (P19)

Overall, the PA intervention was perceived to challenge the balance and stability of most participants.

3.3.2. Comfort of the Exercise Selection

Participants reported their opinions on the comfort of performing the exercises using the elastic resistance band at the hip and chest. This is demonstrated on a level of scaling and by quotes below (Tables 3 and 4):

Table 3. Comfort scores of the exercises performed at the hip region.

Exercise	Hip Region (%)					Mean ± SD Score
	1	2	3	4	5	
Forward step	0	4.3	4.3	13.4	78.0	4.7 ± 0.8
Forward tandem steps	8.6	8.6	13.0	17.4	52.4	4 ± 1.4
Forward tandem hold	8.6	4.3	17.4	4.3	65.4	4.1 ± 1.4
Side steps	0	0	17.4	21.7	60.9	4.4 ± 0.8
Upper body rotation	0	0	4.3	26.2	69.5	4.7 ± 0.6
Backward step	0	0	21.7	26.2	47.8	4.2 ± 0.9
Backward tandem steps	8.6	4.3	17.4	26.2	43.5	3.9 ± 1.3
Backward tandem hold	8.6	0	21.8	21.8	47.8	4 ± 1.2

Notes: Score = percentage score out of 23 participants on a likert scale of 1–5, 1 being very uncomfortable and 5 being very comfortable. Average values presented as mean ± standard deviation.

Table 4. Comfort scores of the exercises performed at the chest region.

Exercise	Chest Region (%)					Mean ± SD Score
	1	2	3	4	5	
Forward step	4.3	4.3	4.3	26.2	60.9	4.3 ± 1.1
Forward tandem steps	8.6	8.6	8.6	26.2	48	4 ± 1.3
Forward tandem hold	8.6	4.3	13.1	21.7	52.3	4 ± 1.3
Side steps	8.6	4.3	0	30.4	56.7	4.2 ± 1.2
Upper body rotation	4.3	4.3	0	26.2	65.2	4.4 ± 1
Backward step	4.3	4.3	8.6	26.2	56.6	4.3 ± 1.1
Backward tandem steps	13	8.6	4.3	26.2	46.9	3.9 ± 1.3
Backward tandem hold	13	4.3	8.6	21.7	52.4	4 ± 1.4

Notes: Score = percentage score out of 23 participants on a likert scale of 1–5, 1 being very uncomfortable and 5 being very comfortable. Average values presented as mean ± standard deviation.

- "It was the effect of the toe to heel and holding that position (tandem steps and tandem holds). It was according to question my ability to hold that position heel to toe. My balance didn't seem to be adequate. I felt less balanced doing them". (P1)
- "I think going backwards if I'm honest, it's a cognitive thing, thinking about going backwards with resistance band type harness on feels slightly less comfortable". (P15)

Furthermore, holding the arms out to the sides during the exercises was an element of the exercises that participants felt was uncomfortable:

- "The only slight issue was that my arms got slightly tired after being held out for as long as it took; but not really an issue". (P18)

- "When you've got the arms out there, we did a number of repetitive ones (exercises) and the upper arms here were starting to ache. So, whether you can reduce that by spreading it around a bit so you're not you're not doing repetitive ones of that. It's not, you know, it's not painful". (P23)

The comfort of the exercises in the intervention was also associated with a perception of enjoyment, the ability to perform the exercises, and a sense of security, which was reported by participants:

- "Yeah, they were all comfortable actually. I enjoyed it a lot really". (P12)
- "It's not physically uncomfortable, none of them were physically uncomfortable. It just felt a lot a lot more secure while doing it" (exercises in the forward direction) (P19)

3.3.3. Preference for the Exercise Selection

Personal preferences for the exercises that were selected were reported by participants on a level of scaling and quotes. (Tables 5 and 6):

Table 5. Enjoyment scores of the exercises performed at the hip region.

Exercise	Hip Region (%)					Mean ± SD Score
	1	2	3	4	5	
Forward step	0	4.3	4.3	17.4	74	4.6 ± 0.8
Forward tandem steps	13	0	13	13	61	4.1 ± 1.4
Forward tandem hold	13	0	8.6	13	65.4	4.2 ± 1.4
Side steps	0	4.3	4.3	34.8	56.6	4.4 ± 0.8
Upper body rotation	0	0	8.6	17.4	74	4.7 ± 0.6
Backward step	4.3	4.3	8.6	26.2	56.6	4.3 ± 1.1
Backward tandem steps	8.6	0	13	17.4	61	4.2 ± 1.2
Backward tandem hold	8.6	0	8.6	21.8	61	4.3 ± 1.2

Notes: Score = percentage score out of 23 participants on a likert scale of 1–5, 1 being not enjoyable and 5 being very enjoyable. Average values presented as mean ± standard deviation.

Table 6. Enjoyment scores of the exercises performed at the chest region.

Exercise	Chest Region (%)					Mean ± SD Score
	1	2	3	4	5	
Forward step	4.3	0	4.3	30.4	61	4.4 ± 0.9
Forward tandem steps	13	0	4.3	30.4	52.3	4.1 ± 1.3
Forward tandem hold	13	0	0	34.8	52.2	4.1 ± 1.3
Side steps	4.3	0	0	30.4	65.3	4.5 ± 0.9
Upper body rotation	4.3	4.3	0	21.7	69.7	4.5 ± 1
Backward step	4.3	0	0	30.4	65.2	4.5 ± 0.9
Backward tandem steps	13	0	4.3	26.1	56.6	4.1 ± 1.4
Backward tandem hold	13	0	0	30.4	56.6	4.2 ± 1.3

Notes: Score = percentage score out of 23 participants on a likert scale of 1–5, 1 being not enjoyable and 5 being very enjoyable. Average values presented as mean ± standard deviation.

The participants reported their preference for the exercise selection:

- Forward step: "Personal favourite, I think. But I found that it's not too hard, so that's the reason why I'm saying it isn't it, but I think that these ones the tandem ones, balancing ones I like them as well because I feel that it's challenging you. So, I have to say that I think that they are probably the most beneficial out of all of them. I quite like that one backwards (backward tandem steps) that challenges you backwards". (P4)
- "I like the side steps because I felt it on my sides, and I thought that is really good. I did like this (tandem holds) because I was pushing and then I felt it in my arms as well. I liked the twist (upper body rotations)—for me the release of my back muscles really". (P11)

Several participants reported what they disliked about the exercises:

- "The only ones I didn't like was the placement of the feet one in front of the other (tandem holds) and having to hold. It's the balance aspect". (P1)

- "The parallel steps or the little fairy steps (tandem steps) or whatever they are called I definitely didn't, but again, it may well be doing you very good". (P19)
- "Probably one I disliked was the sides the side steps only on the left-hand side. I had to step back with my left foot. I found out my left side is my weaker side anyway, so it's even proved it even more now so". (P21)

Performing exercises backwards was highlighted as the least favourite exercise of participants:

- "I'm okay with the backward ones. It's just that you can't see behind you. It can be a bit disconcerting. I wouldn't say I dislike them, but you know, if I didn't have to do it then I wouldn't bother doing it". (P3)
- "Backward steps, they were difficult again for not seeing. And then the tandem one I couldn't do that at all anyway". (P6)

3.3.4. Difficulty of the Exercise Selection

Participants reported their opinions on the difficulty of performing the exercises using the elastic resistance band around the hip and chest. This is demonstrated on a level of scaling and by the quotes below (Tables 7 and 8):

Table 7. Difficulty scores of the exercises performed at the hip region.

Exercise	Hip Region (%)					Mean ± SD Score
	1	2	3	4	5	
Forward step	0	0	13	21.7	65.3	4.5 ± 0.7
Forward tandem steps	4.3	8.6	30.4	30.4	26.3	3.7 ± 1.1
Forward tandem hold	4.3	17.4	13	43.5	21.8	3.6 ± 1.2
Side steps	4.3	4.3	4.3	26.1	61	4.3 ± 1.1
Upper body rotation	0	4.3	8.6	7.4	69.7	4.5 ± 0.8
Backward step	0	8.6	8.6	26.1	56.7	4.3 ± 1
Backward tandem steps	8.6	4.3	21.7	43.5	21.9	3.7 ± 1.2
Backward tandem hold	8.6	8.6	13	43.5	26.3	3.7 ± 1.2

Notes: Score = percentage score out of 23 participants on a likert scale of 1–5, 1 being extremely difficult and 5 being extremely easy to perform. Average values presented as mean ± standard deviation.

Table 8. Enjoyment scores of the exercises performed at the hip region.

Exercise	Chest Region (%)					Mean ± SD Score
	1	2	3	4	5	
Forward step	4.3	0	0	26.1	69.6	4.6 ± 0.9
Forward tandem steps	4.3	8.6	17.4	30.4	39.3	3.9 ± 1.2
Forward tandem hold	4.3	8.6	17.4	30.4	39.3	3.9 ± 1.2
Side steps	4.3	4.3	4.3	34.8	52.3	4.3 ± 1.1
Upper body rotation	0	4.3	8.6	17.4	69.7	4.5 ± 0.8
Backward step	0	4.3	13	30.4	52.3	4.3 ± 0.9
Backward tandem steps	8.6	4.3	21.7	34.8	30.6	3.7 ± 1.2
Backward tandem hold	8.6	4.3	21.7	34.8	30.6	3.7 ± 1.2

Notes: Score = percentage score out of 23 participants on a likert scale of 1–5, 1 being extremely difficult and 5 being extremely easy to perform. Average values presented as mean ± standard deviation.

- "I found them [the exercises] difficult, challenging to do not the end of the world thing but just felt a little bit challenging. It's just the balance I guess, which I know is the object to this in a lot of ways. But as I say, they're harder (tandem steps), but maybe in terms of this whole thing they become very important". (P19)
- Tandem steps and tandem holds: "I think anything to do with like the balance is harder, but it's supposed to be right? It's challenging more than just stepping forward, it is challenging new balance, isn't it?". (P4)

In other cases, participants did not perceive the exercises to be difficult to perform:

- "There aren't too tough and definitely weren't too easy, and I wouldn't even say they were too tough". (P2)

- "I don't think any of them seemed really difficult. I would say it was quite easy to do them once I got my head in mind with what I'm supposed to be doing. I didn't find them difficult, any of them difficult". (P15)

3.3.5. Heart Rate and RPE Measures

The two-way mixed model ANOVA revealed a significant main effect of time ($F = 60.888$, $p < 0.001$, $\eta_p^2 = 0.74$) but not condition ($F = 3.567$, $p = 0.07$, $\eta_p^2 = 0.14$) for HR. Post hoc within-subject analyses revealed significant ($p < 0.01$) increases in HR from pre- to mid- to post-intervention in hip (pre- = 85 ± 11 bpm, mid- = 88 ± 11 bpm, post-intervention 89 = ± 11 bpm, 5%) and chest (pre- = 83 ± 12 bpm, mid- = 85 ± 12 bpm, post-intervention = 88 ± 12 bpm, 6%) conditions (Figure 4).

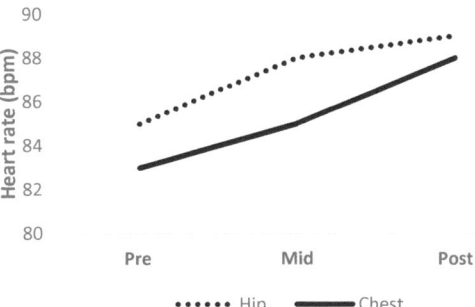

Figure 4. Heart rates measured at pre-, mid-, and post-intervention with the elastic band placed at the hip (dotted line) and chest (solid line).

The two-way mixed model ANOVA revealed a significant main effect of time ($F = 23.433$, $p < 0.001$, $\eta_p^2 = 0.52$) but not condition ($F = 3.477$, $p = 0.08$, $\eta_p^2 = 0.14$) for RPE. Post hoc within-subject analyses revealed significant ($p < 0.05$) increases in RPE from pre- to mid- to post-intervention in hip (pre- = 8 ± 2, mid- = 10 ± 2, post-intervention = 10 ± 2) and chest (pre- = 9 ± 2, mid- = 10 ± 2, post-intervention = 11 ± 2) conditions (Figure 5).

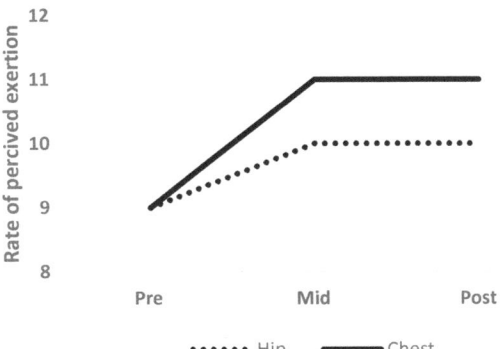

Figure 5. Rate of perceived exertion measured at pre-, mid-, and post-intervention with the elastic band placed at the hip (dotted line) and chest (solid line).

3.3.6. Organisation of the Exercise Selection

Participants reported on the way that the exercises were organised. The repetitions and sets of exercises were perceived to be adequate. Participant responses were as follows:
- "I thought that was adequate. No, I don't think you could delete any of those and I can't think of anything that you could add". (P1)

- "I think that was ample. Yeah, that was ample to do that was just a right level from my perspective as a person, it was right for me". (P3)

However, in some cases, participants felt that the repetitions and sets of exercises could have been increased.

- "I think for me I could have done more repetitions, um, but again that would have to be assessed depending on each individual". (P11)
- "It was just starting to make me get into that zone. For others, I can imagine that being too much and for others again who are at the fitter end of the spectrum wouldn't have found the earlier ones (exercises) particularly demanding". (P20)

3.3.7. Suitability of the PA Intervention

Participants discussed their personal views on how the PA intervention was suitable for themselves and other people within their age group:

- "I would have thought so, yes. I mean, everybody is individual". (P8)
- "Yes, it's a good idea because balance is our main problem as we get older". (P14)

In some cases, participants felt the exercises were not age-appropriate:

- "No, I don't. I don't know really because I don't find them particularly difficult, but I can imagine somebody who's not used to it, because I do other things. I wouldn't know if anybody else would find them difficult. Yeah, that all depends on the level of ability really doesn't it really". (P9)
- "For me, not particularly, but I can imagine if I give it 10 years, well, hopefully 20 years they will be". (P18)

3.3.8. Perceived benefits of the PA intervention

Participants discussed why they felt the exercises were beneficial, as illustrated in the following cases:

- "I just think they give a good workout on the hips and the legs and the knees. I can see the benefits of that, you know". (P3)
- "They might very well be doing you a lot of good, particularly the side (side steps). I don't know what it is, but there is something about that I just feel I ought to do that more. I don't know, just something about that exercise that just feels as though it's doing me good, without being painful. It feels like something that you ought to include in regular exercise". (P19)

3.3.9. The Psychosocial Impact of the PA Intervention

Participants discussed the psychosocial impacts of the PA intervention. In particular, participants discussed their level of confidence in performing the exercises:

- "It's confidence, it's your confidence knowing you can do it" (P13)
- "I think it's a confidence thing with where you're putting your feet as well. How far I felt I could put my feet forward or backward depending on which exercise I was doing and how hard I was pushing against the bands". (P15)

Participants reported if anxiousness was an aspect that they experienced when performing the exercises (Supplementary File S2).

Participants reported if the exercises made them focus their attention on the task at hand:

- "I thought the others were good because they were challenging and you had to stay focused, particularly number two and three (tandem steps and tandem hold) you had stay focused". (P11)
- "I was probably flagging a little bit in terms of concentration, not in terms of physical energy, but I think you know after a bit when you've been doing things that you have to really think about what you're doing a bit harder". (P15)

All the participants reported a positive experience regarding their participation and that they would perform the exercises again (Supplementary File S2).

3.4. Opinions of the Exercise Equipment

3.4.1. Preferences for the Elastic Band Placement

Participants reported what they specifically liked about performing the exercises with the elastic band placed at the hip:

- "I could feel the tug when It was on the hips, you know, so I knew I was working extra hard with it on the hips". (P3)
- "I think it's the right tension" (P9)

The participants reported their opinions on the safety aspect and what they liked about performing the exercises with the elastic band placed at the chest:

- "I think it's the right tension" (P9)
- "I thought the harness work very well indeed. In all of them. I just felt better with it like that than I did in the hip position. I did prefer the harness a lot but particularly when you were facing away from the anchor". (P19)

Furthermore, participants discussed what they disliked about performing the exercises with the elastic band placed at the hip:

- "My thing is just about the band not having the stability on the first lot of exercises, whereas with the harness [chest region] you've got more of the stability because I think it detracts from your concentration of what you're doing". (P3)
- "You don't seem to have support with the hip one. It can slip at any time. I've got love handles so it sits on me but for somebody who hasn't got enough I imagine it's very hard". (P6)

Participants also stated what they disliked about the chest:

- "I think it was just uncomfortable. It wasn't the exercises, it was just the feeling of. It being uncomfortable". (P4)
- "It was a bit restricted on the chest. It wasn't so enjoyable as with the bottom one". (P6)

In some cases, female participants reported how they felt restricted wearing the chest harness equipment with the elastic band placed at the chest (Supplementary File S2).

3.4.2. Difficulty of Exercises Performed with the Elastic Band Placed at the Hip

The difficulty of performing the exercises was further discussed in terms of the elastic band placement:

Hip Region (Figure 1).

- "It was difficult at the hip. You've got more support with the chest one". (P6) "With it round your hips I found more challenging. I felt as if I was going to get pinged back". (P7)
- "It was more challenging to use center of balance and more around your center [hip region] than on top where you can lean into it, if you know what I mean. You can't use your body weight on it. It's more attacking your balance from your hips". (P21)

Chest Region (Figure 1).

- "Chest, I just felt there's more resistance". (P18)
- "With your upper half you've got the whole of your body, whereas with your lower half you're using your bottom part, so I've found it easier with the whole of my body [chest region]. If you're pushing something, you push it with the whole of your body so it's easier, isn't it?". (P11)

3.4.3. Preferred Elastic Band Placement

Participants' preference for their preferred elastic band location while performing the exercises was reported. This is demonstrated in the table and quotes below (Table 9).

Table 9. Participants' preferences for the location of the elastic band.

Preference	Elastic Band Placement (*n* = 23)		
	Chest	Hip	Either
To perform again	11	7	5
Safety	12	7	4

Notes: chest: elastic band placed at the chest region. Hip: elastic band placed at the hip region and either: Participants did not have a preferred placement of the elastic band.

- "It just depends on the equipment whether there is a different form, a different way that you could do the hip one. It would probably be the hip one if there was a change". (P6)
- "I don't have a problem providing somebody can come up with a solution involved in the band around the waist (hip region). I could feel it slipping so that it that was a bit of an issue I suppose". (P22)

The safety element in terms of the exercise equipment was an aspect reported by participants with the elastic band placed at the chest (Table 6), which they felt provided a greater sense of safety.

- "Chest, only that the Velcro seemed to hold better there than at the hip". (P1)
- "Safer, definitely with the chest harness on". (P5)
- "I don't think there was any difference for me. I think that I felt okay at either". (P11)

3.5. Environment

Supervision, clear verbal instruction on how to perform the exercises, and a safety briefing on the exercise equipment were factors reported to help to create a sense of a safe environment (Supplementary File S2).

3.5.1. Safety Factors

- "Just realising the band was holding and having you three around me". (P8)
- "I knew what to expect because you had explained to me about the bands, so I was fully informed, you created a safe environment". (P2)
- "I know you were there. I trusted you that it's hooked into the ground, so that's fine. It's not going to come out". (P12)

3.5.2. Preferred Setting

Performing the exercises in a supervised/group setting was preferred by participants.

- "I'd prefer a group setting. Fellow participants would encourage each other. There'd be the social aspect because there'd be an interchange of conversations, whereas. If you're on your own there wouldn't". (P1)
- "My preference would be with other individuals or certainly with an instructor". (P23)

3.5.3. Shaping the PA Intervention

Participants provided their own ideas about how the intervention design could be shaped, including aspects that could be done differently.

Equipment:

- "I think the band would be better hugging the hip a bit. It could mould itself more into the hip than that then it won't be sliding down the leg". (P3)
- "If you had a belt that you could strap round to whatever size you want your body was and had two little clips on the side which fit to the band". (P6)
- "I think if it were a little bit wider (the elastic band) it might be a little bit more comfortable". (P9)
- "I would suggest doing it at the side of the hips so that you've got an anchor point for front and rear, so they somehow have a pully up or anything like that they are going to feel uncomfortable because it's actually pulling on part of the body". (P21)

- "Another belt with it like one that does the weightlifting sticks of Velcro on that using one of them". (P22)
- "Whether you could adapt a system around your waist which will actually take this the slippage away, that would help". (P23)

Adaptations:

- "Incorporate more things like a weight". (P5)
- "What might have been good is if you've got like your line which you have over there (marker on the ground) then you've got different markers. So, you've got a progression in your mind". (P11)
- "I think the other thing is to apply this to different activities or something like that will also help". (P12)
- "I guess you could even do like a circuit, you know where you go from each one in turn and then go through them again". (P19)
- "So, it incorporates it so it's a bit more of a program almost. Little lunges that's sort of thing. What we do we always try to do a warmup then a workout and then a warm down". (P20)
- "Whether you could think about introducing a stronger band, I don't know. When you're doing the same band, it's going to get to get monotonous because I'm going to find it easier and easier and easier". (P22)

4. Discussion

In the current study, the feasibility of a novel PA intervention using elastic band resistance at the hip and chest to challenge balance in older adults was evaluated. The study was designed to include multiple data sets to inform the design of the PA intervention by using interviews to investigate their personal preferences, difficulty, comfort, suitability, perceived benefits, safety, exercise equipment, and the environment. Additionally, quantitative data of HR and RPE were used to determine the PA intensity. These multiple data sets were combined with the feedback from older adults as a unique aspect to the study, which contributes to informing the process of designing PA interventions that are feasible for older adults [1,32,33]. The benefits of involving older adults in the development of such interventions has been shown to encourage older adults to be physically active [34].

The present study identified the feasibility of a novel elastic band resistance PA intervention and the importance of delivery to make older adults feel comfortable and safe, including a sense of enjoyment and considering the environment as well as the preferences and physical abilities of each individual. Therefore, it is important to discuss the outcomes of the study, which include considerations that may be useful for future PA interventions to meet the needs of older adults.

4.1. Perceptions of the Exercises

Participants varied in their perceptions of how challenging the PA intervention was regarding balance. However, exercises including the upper-body rotations and the side steps were perceived to be less challenging. These exercises were performed with a wider base of support, which is a likely explanation for the greater stability experienced, influencing participants' perception that they insufficiently challenged balance [35].

In terms of difficulty, participants suggested that the chest exercises were easier to perform as they could use the force of their whole body to lean against the resistance band to maintain balance, whereas hip exercises were restricted to using the force of the lower body only and were perceived to be more difficult. Furthermore, this may be due to activation of additional muscles, including those in the trunk/core area, which may provide greater benefit to balance performance compared to hip exercises [36].

Holding the arms out to each side of the body during the tandem exercises (Figure 1 (Images 2,3,7,8)) was perceived to increase exercise difficulty. This may be due to the additional cognitive demand of performing two tasks simultaneously, requiring greater coordination [36]. Previous studies have highlighted an increase in perceived difficulty in dual-task exercises and a decrease in balance performance [37–39]. Providing the option of a dual-task element in the PA intervention would therefore provide an additional challenge to increase difficulty for people who require it, allowing greater individualisation of the training prescription and potentially improving intervention effectiveness.

4.1.1. Perceptions of Age and Balance Capacity

According to the verbal feedback, participants who perceived themselves to be older also tended to view their balance as poorer (Section 3.3.4, Section 3.3.6). As ageing is associated with a reduction in physical function, including reduced muscle strength, coordination, and balance [40], this is likely explained by age-related fear of falling [41,42].

4.1.2. Psychological and Motivational Considerations

The participants' perception of their ability to perform the exercises was related to confidence, self-efficacy, and comfort (Section 3.3.9), which are determinants of PA for older adults [43]. Participants expressed that they felt less comfortable performing the exercises that most challenged balance (i.e., tandem steps, tandem holds, and performed exercises backwards), and this likely placed increased demand on postural control and coordination due to the narrow base of support. Most participants did not report anxiousness whilst performing the exercises, possibly due to the close supervision by staff, with whom the participants were well-acquainted [44]. Furthermore, other factors that likely contributed to participants' confidence levels were the clear verbal instruction for how to perform the exercises and a detailed safety briefing on the PA equipment to provide everyone with the confidence to perform the exercises (Section 3.5.1). Previous research has highlighted benefits of providing both verbal and written instructions to increase compliance and motivation regarding PA in younger adults [44,45], which provides a sense of security and safety during the intervention. The current intervention considered this aspect within the design with older adults and highlighted the importance of this aspect when creating PA interventions for this age group.

4.1.3. Perceptions of the Elastic Band Placement

Participants perceived the chest placement of the elastic band to provide a greater sense of security in terms of safety whilst performing the exercises compared to the hip placement. This perception may be related to the points addressed previously with the chest intervention being less challenging in terms of the balance required to perform the exercises compared to that with band placement at the hip. Sex was a factor associated with the perceived comfort of the exercise selection, with females expressing how the chest harness felt uncomfortable due to the placement of the elastic band high on the anatomical position of the chest, whereas this was not a concern for males. This suggests that the chest intervention may not be feasible, or at least less preferred, than the hip intervention for some females. Regardless, both locations of the elastic band placement (chest and hip) were reported to be challenging with regard to balance. Thus, the exercise equipment and the elastic band placement should be taken into consideration or be modified to suit individuals in future interventions.

4.1.4. Perceptions of Intervention

The personal preferences reported for the exercise selection were associated with the ability to perform the exercises, with participants preferring to perform the exercises that were less difficult and at which they therefore felt more capable and confident to perform. This ease provided participants with a greater sense of enjoyment due to being able to perform the selected exercises [46]. The importance of enjoyment in PA is recognised as an essential aspect of engagement for older adults, which should be considered in PA interventions for older adults [46]. Additionally, enjoyment is highlighted in the SEM as a factor that makes activities accessible and appealing [7]. The PA interventions have the potential to provide a graded challenge to allow individuals to become proficient and efficacious in the exercises over time, which has previously been highlighted as a motivational factor, and should thus be considered for older adults [44].

4.1.5. Perceptions of Exercise Intensity

The PA intervention was delivered at a low/moderate intensity, which can be altered to gradually increase the intensity over time to provide a continuously challenging program as the neuromuscular system adapts [47]. The adaptability of the exercises would allow participants to progress at their own pace with the activity, which has been highlighted as an important aspect in engaging older adults in PA within the SEM [7,48]. Including this aspect of adaptability in PA interventions for older adults enables individuals with varying needs to participate in PA and allows older adults to exercise within the limits of their own abilities [44].

4.1.6. Exercise Intensity: Heart Rate (HR) and Perceived Exertion (RPE)

Heart rate and RPE measures indicated that the intensity of the PA intervention increased to a low-to-moderate level. Although moderate-to-vigorous levels of PA are recommended in the PA guidelines for older adults [16], the physical and mental health benefits of increasing sedentary levels of PA may be overlooked. The importance of providing older adults with the confidence to engage in PA to be more active is essential to promote behaviour changes and leads to increased PA levels over time [44,45]. The current PA interventions can be tailored for varying physical abilities and can be modified to increase the difficulty and therefore intensity of the exercises over time to meet individual needs.

4.1.7. Reflection on Aspects of Socialisation

Within this study, all participants reported a positive experience from engaging in the PA. A contributing factor was the social interaction aspect, which emerged as a general theme (Section 3.5.2). The interaction with the researchers/supervisors was a facilitator of engagement in the intervention. The importance of the social element has previously been identified in the self-determination theory [10,11] as a facilitator that motivates behaviour, which may promote behaviour change in PA engagement [49]. A prominent theme was that the group setting/supervision was the preferred environment of participants to engage and perform the PA intervention, which is consistent with previous research indicating the importance of the social aspect in providing participants with motivation, enjoyment, and social interaction. Other studies have shown that theses aspects are important factors to be considered in PA interventions to make them appealing and engaging for older adults [50]. The SEM demonstrates the importance of this social element in activities as an essential motivator for older adults to adhere to PA [7]. Furthermore, as this research was conducted during COVID-19 restrictions, group contact may have been a concern. However, some of the participants wanted the group contact, which may explain the personal preference for a preferred group setting [27]. As older adults may be at high risk of social isolation [51], the opportunity for social engagement is an important aspect to be considered in PA interventions to influence relationships and improve social connectedness to provide a positive experience [52]. Future considerations of a group setting for the current PA interventions would be advantageous to make the intervention accessible for older adults [7,53].

4.1.8. Organisation and Tailoring

The opinion about the exercise organisation in terms of the sets and repetitions varied for each participant. This was likely a result of each participants' previous experience of PA [44]. This further enhances the importance of individual tailoring and meeting individual needs, which has previously been stated to be a safe and effective approach to improving physical outcomes in older adults [54,55]. The perceived suitability of the intervention was considered to ensure that the intervention was suitable for older adults. Participants revealed that they felt the intervention was suitable for themselves and others in their age group as they were aware of the deterioration of balance control in ageing. The participants in the older age group (65–84 years) reported perceived benefits of performing the exercises, associated with their own abilities to perform the exercises. However, participants in the younger age bracket (50–64 years) thought that the exercises would be beneficial at a later age when their balance control would be decreased, although at this age (50–64 years), this could possibly be considered as too late. Providing the opportunity for an early preventative PA intervention in middle-aged adults to improve and maintain balance performance may be key to delaying declines in daily functioning and falls later in life [56,57].

Importantly, the opinions and ideas of older adults have contributed to shaping the design of the intervention. This included ways in which the equipment can be altered to provide comfort and ways to progress the intervention to make it more challenging, such as incorporating weights, incorporating the exercises in a multicomponent intervention, and increasing the resistance of the elastic band to further challenge balance. The inclusion of progressively challenging balancing exercises is essential in such interventions as the body's sensory systems are highly adaptive [58]. Modifications should be considered to suit individual preferences in PA interventions for older adults, for example, by altering the resistance of the elastic band and having participants stand out further from the anchor point to increase the resistance and instability and therefore make the exercises progressively more challenging to improve and adapt balance control strategies [59]. The practice of postural control strategies helps to improve and challenge balance, supporting the ideology of the PA intervention [35].

4.2. Strengths and Limitations

An important strength of the present study is that it provided rich information about the perceptions of the PA design of older adults and utilised the participants' perceptions/feedback to shape the intervention. This is useful for directing future PA interventions for older adults to make them accessible, enjoyable, and appropriate. Further, the present study shares the process of how to undertake this research, involving older adults in the development of shaping and designing interventions to meet their needs, as called for in the literature [7]. This will be helpful for other stakeholders seeking to identify the preferences for the exercise section, safety, social, and enjoyment factors. These research findings will be disseminated to older adults and the providers of services for older adults through local PA networks in Derbyshire and the East Midlands (UK). Furthermore, whilst this study evaluated the perceptions of older adults, participants' balance performances were not measured directly using a balance performance measure. This research was conducted during COVID-19 restrictions with safety precautions, although the recruitment to the study was limited to those individuals who felt confident in the university setting during this time.

5. Conclusions

In this study, the insights, opinions, and preferences regarding the novel **elastic** band resistance PA protocol provided valuable information for designing and shaping future PA interventions suitable for older adults. The importance of including security, safety, and the option of regressions and progressions in PA tailored to individual needs/abilities should be considered within such interventions. The enjoyment, socialisation, and perceived benefits of performing PA are important aspects and motivating factors in older adults' decision to engage in PA. Given the outcomes, it would suggest that the PA intervention is feasible and appropriate for **older adults** to perform at a low-to-moderate exercise intensity. Ongoing efforts to involve and include older adults in the intervention design to meet the needs and preferences of older adults are of significance to enable PA interventions to be successful. This study contributes to the development of a novel PA intervention using elastic band resistance training to challenge balance and utilised the perspectives of **older adults** in shaping an accessible, appropriate, and acceptable intervention to meet their needs. Furthermore, the current intervention has the potential to improve balance in **older adults** and therefore prevent falls and mitigate fall occurrences, although further research is required to identify the effects on balance and postural sway patterns to confirm the efficacy of the program in mitigating common fall risk characteristics.

Supplementary Materials: The following supporting information can be downloaded at: https://www.mdpi.com/article/10.3390/ijerph191710907/s1, Supplementary File S1: Refinement of methods during piloting; Supplementary File S2: Quotations from interview schedules.

Author Contributions: Conceptualisation, N.M.D., A.P., A.D.K., M.A.F., A.J.B. and M.A.M.; Methodology, N.M.D., A.P., A.D.K., A.J.B. and M.A.M.; Formal Analysis, N.M.D., A.P., A.D.K. and M.A.M.; Investigation, N.M.D. and D.T.; Data Curation, N.M.D. and D.T.; Writing—Original Draft Preparation, N.M.D., A.P., A.D.K., A.J.B. and M.A.M.; Writing—Review and Editing, N.M.D., A.P., A.D.K., A.J.B. and M.A.M.; Supervision, A.P., A.D.K., M.A.F., A.J.B. and M.A.M.; Funding Acquisition, N.M.D. All authors have read and agreed to the published version of the manuscript.

Funding: This research received no external funding.

Institutional Review Board Statement: The study was conducted according to the guidelines of the Declaration of Helsinki and was reviewed and approved by University of Derby, College of Science and Engineering (ID: ETH2021/4503, 21 July 2021).

Informed Consent Statement: Informed consent was obtained from all subjects involved in the study.

Data Availability Statement: The data are not publicly available due to ethical restrictions. Please contact the corresponding author for further information.

Acknowledgments: The authors would like to acknowledge all of the participants that contributed and gave their time to take part in the research study. Thank you to all of the university laboratory technicians for their support.

Conflicts of Interest: The authors declare no conflict of interest.

References

1. Government. 2022. Available online: https://www.gov.uk/government/publications/falls-applying-all-our-health/falls-applying-all-our-health (accessed on 18 April 2022).
2. National Health Service (NHS). 2019. Available online: https://www.nhs.uk/conditions/Falls/ (accessed on 2 November 2019).
3. Fang, Q.; Ghanouni, P.; Anderson, S.E.; Touchett, H.; Shirley, R.; Fang, F.; Fang, C. Effects of exergaming on balance of healthy older adults: A systematic review and meta-analysis of randomized controlled trials. *Games Health J.* **2020**, *9*, 11–23. [CrossRef] [PubMed]
4. Shumway-Cook, A.; Woollacott, M.H. *Motor Control: Translating Research into Clinical Practice*, 5th ed.; Lippincott Williams & Wilkins: Philadelphia, PA, USA, 2017.
5. Kim, Y.; Vakula, M.N.; Bolton, D.A.; Dakin, C.J.; Thompson, B.J.; Slocum, T.A.; Teramoto, M.; Bressel, E. Which Exercise Interventions Can Most Effectively Improve Reactive Balance in Older Adults? A Systematic Review and Network Meta-Analysis. *Front. Aging Neurosci.* **2022**, *13*, 992. [CrossRef] [PubMed]
6. Gerards, M.H.; McCrum, C.; Mansfield, A.; Meijer, K. Perturbation-based balance training for falls reduction among older adults: Current evidence and implications for clinical practice. *Geriatr. Gerontol. Int.* **2017**, *17*, 2294–2303. [CrossRef] [PubMed]
7. Boulton, E.R.; Horne, M.; Todd, C. Multiple influences on participating in physical activity in older age: Developing a social ecological approach. *Health Expect.* **2018**, *21*, 239–248. [CrossRef]
8. Teixeira, P.J.; Carraça, E.V.; Markland, D.; Silva, M.N.; Ryan, R.M. Exercise, physical activity, and self-determination theory: A systematic review. *Int. J. Behav. Nutr. Phys. Act.* **2012**, *9*, 78. [CrossRef]
9. Deci, E.L.; Ryan, R.M. The" what" and" why" of goal pursuits: Human needs and the self-determination of behavior. *Psychol. Inq.* **2000**, *11*, 227–268. [CrossRef]
10. Moore, B.M.; Adams, J.T.; Willcox, S.; Nicholson, J. The effect of active physical training interventions on reactive postural responses in older adults: A systematic review. *J. Aging Phys. Act.* **2019**, *27*, 252–264. [CrossRef]
11. Grabiner, M.D.; Bareither, M.L.; Gatts, S.; Marone, J.; Troy, K.L. Task-specific training reduces trip-related fall risk in women. *Med. Sci. Sports Exerc.* **2012**, *44*, 2410–2414. [CrossRef]
12. Kurz, I.; Gimmon, Y.; Shapiro, A.; Debi, R.; Snir, Y.; Melzer, I. Unexpected perturbations training improves balance control and voluntary stepping times in older adults-a double blind randomized control trial. *BMC Geriatr.* **2016**, *16*, 58. [CrossRef]
13. Pai, Y.C.; Bhatt, T.; Yang, F.; Wang, E.; Kritchevsky, S. Perturbation training can reduce community-dwelling older adults' annual fall risk: A randomized controlled trial. *J. Gerontol. Ser. A Biomed. Sci. Med. Sci.* **2014**, *69*, 1586–1594. [CrossRef]

14. Paquette, M.R.; Li, Y.; Hoekstra, J.; Bravo, J. An 8-week reactive balance training program in older healthy adults: A preliminary investigation. *J. Sport Health Sci.* **2015**, *4*, 263–269. [CrossRef]
15. Mansfield, A.; Wong, J.S.; Bryce, J.; Knorr, S.; Patterson, K.K. Does perturbation-based balance training prevent falls? Systematic review and meta-analysis of preliminary randomized controlled trials. *Phys. Ther.* **2015**, *95*, 700–709. [CrossRef]
16. Physical Activity Guidelines: UK Chief Medical Officers' Report. 2022. Available online: https://www.gov.uk/government/publications/physical-activity-guidelines-uk-chief-medical-officers-report (accessed on 29 May 2022).
17. Lima, F.F.; Camillo, C.A.; Gobbo, L.A.; Trevisan, I.B.; Nascimento, W.B.; Silva, B.S.; Lima, M.C.S.; Ramos, D.; Ramos, E.M. Resistance training using low cost elastic tubing is equally effective to conventional weight machines in middle-aged to older healthy adults: A quasi-randomized controlled clinical trial. *J. Sports Sci. Med.* **2018**, *17*, 153.
18. Behm, D.G. An analysis of intermediate speed resistance exercises for velocity-specific strength gains. *J. Appl. Sport Sci. Res.* **1991**, *5*, 1–5.
19. Colado, J.C.; García-Massó, X.; Pellicer, M.; Alakhdar, Y.; Benavent, J.; Cabeza-Ruiz, R. A comparison of elastic tubing and isotonic resistance exercises. *Int. J. Sports Med.* **2010**, *31*, 810–817. [CrossRef]
20. Colado, J.C.; Triplett, N.T. Effects of a short-term resistance program using elastic bands versus weight machines for sedentary middle-aged women. *J. Strength Cond. Res.* **2008**, *22*, 1441–1448. [CrossRef] [PubMed]
21. Rogers, M.E.; Page, P.; Takeshima, N. Balance training for the older athlete. *Int. J. Sports Phys. Ther.* **2013**, *8*, 517. [PubMed]
22. Kocaogly, Y.; Erkmen, N. The Effect of Elastic Resistance Band Training on Postural Control and Body Composition in Sedentary Women. *Spor. Bilimleri. Araştırmaları. Derg.* **2021**, *6*, 233–245. [CrossRef]
23. Yeun, Y.R. Effectiveness of resistance exercise using elastic bands on flexibility and balance among the elderly people living in the community: A systematic review and meta-analysis. *J. Phys. Ther. Sci.* **2017**, *29*, 1695–1699. [CrossRef]
24. Kwak, C.J.; Kim, Y.L.; Lee, S.M. Effects of elastic-band resistance exercise on balance, mobility and gait function, flexibility and fall efficacy in elderly people. *J. Phys. Ther. Sci.* **2016**, *28*, 3189–3196. [CrossRef]
25. Leask, C.F.; Colledge, N.; Laventure, R.M.; McCann, D.A.; Skelton, D.A. Co-creating recommendations to redesign and promote strength and balance service provision. *Int. J. Environ. Res. Public Health* **2019**, *16*, 3169. [CrossRef] [PubMed]
26. Kime, N.; Pringle, A.; Zwolinsky, S.; Vishnubala, D. How prepared are healthcare professionals for delivering physical activity guidance to those with diabetes? A formative evaluation. *BMC Health Serv. Res.* **2020**, *20*, 8. [CrossRef] [PubMed]
27. Lozano-Sufrategui, L.; Pringle, A.; Zwolinsky, S.; Drew, K.J. Professional football clubs' involvement in health promotion in Spain: An audit of current practices. *Health Promot. Int.* **2020**, *35*, 994–1004. [CrossRef] [PubMed]
28. Pringle, A.; Kime, N.; Zwolinsky, S.; Rutherford, Z.; Roscoe, C.M. An Investigation into the Physical Activity Experiences of People Living with and beyond Cancer during the COVID-19 Pandemic. *Int. J. Environ. Res. Public Health* **2022**, *19*, 2945. [CrossRef] [PubMed]
29. King, N. Doing template analysis. *Qual. Organ. Res. Core Methods Curr. Chall.* **2012**, *426*, 77–101.
30. Brooks, J.; McCluskey, S.; Turley, E.; King, N. The utility of template analysis in qualitative psychology research. *Qual. Res. Psychol.* **2015**, *12*, 202–222. [CrossRef]
31. Braun, V.; Clarke, V. Using thematic analysis in psychology. *Qual. Res. Psychol.* **2006**, *3*, 77–101. [CrossRef]
32. Pringle, A.; Zwolinsky, S. Older adults, physical activity and public health. In *Sport and Health: Exploring the Current State of Play*; Routledge: London, UK, 2017; pp. 81–110.
33. Quality Statement 2: Physical Activity for Older People | Mental Wellbeing and Independence for Older People | Quality Standards | NICE. 2016. Available online: https://www.nice.org.uk/guidance/qs137/chapter/quality-statement-2-physical-activity-for-older-people (accessed on 26 April 2022).
34. Boulton, E.R.; Horne, M.; Todd, C. Involving older adults in developing physical activity interventions to promote engagement: A literature review. *J. Popul. Ageing* **2020**, *13*, 325–345. [CrossRef]
35. Howe, T.E.; Rochester, L.; Neil, F.; Skelton, D.A.; Ballinger, C. Exercise for improving balance in older people. *Cochrane Database Syst. Rev.* **2011**, *11*, CD004963. [CrossRef]
36. Haruyama, K.; Kawakami, M.; Otsuka, T. Effect of core stability training on trunk function, standing balance, and mobility in stroke patients: A randomized controlled trial. *Neurorehabil. Neural Repair* **2017**, *31*, 240–249. [CrossRef]
37. Silsupadol, P.; Siu, K.C.; Shumway-Cook, A.; Woollacott, M.H. Training of balance under single-and dual-task conditions in older adults with balance impairment. *Phys. Ther.* **2006**, *86*, 269–281. [CrossRef]
38. Berg, W.P.; Alessio, H.M.; Mills, E.M.; Tong, C. Circumstances and consequences of falls in independent community-dwelling older adults. *Age Ageing* **1997**, *26*, 261–268. [CrossRef] [PubMed]
39. Verghese, J.; Buschke, H.; Viola, L.; Katz, M.; Hall, C.; Kuslansky, G.; Lipton, R. Validity of divided attention tasks in predicting falls in older individuals: A preliminary study. *J. Am. Geriatr. Soc.* **2002**, *50*, 1572–1576. [CrossRef] [PubMed]
40. Kumar, A.; Delbaere, K.; Zijlstra, G.A.R.; Carpenter, H.; Iliffe, S.; Masud, T.; Skelton, D.; Morris, R.; Kendrick, D. Exercise for reducing fear of falling in older people living in the community: Cochrane systematic review and meta-analysis. *Age Ageing* **2016**, *45*, 345–352. [CrossRef] [PubMed]
41. Tinetti, M.E. Performance-oriented assessment of mobility problems in elderly patients. *J. Am. Geriatr. Society* **1986**, *34*, 119–126. [CrossRef]
42. Sapmaz, M.; Mujdeci, B. The effect of fear of falling on balance and dual task performance in the elderly. *Exp. Gerontol.* **2021**, *147*, 111250. [CrossRef]

43. Warner, L.M.; Schüz, B.; Knittle, K.; Ziegelmann, J.P.; Wurm, S. Sources of perceived self-efficacy as predictors of physical activity in older adults. *Appl. Psychol. Health Well-Being* **2011**, *3*, 172–192. [CrossRef]
44. Phillips, E.M.; Schneider, J.C.; Mercer, G.R. Motivating elders to initiate and maintain exercise. *Arch. Phys. Med. Rehabil.* **2004**, *85*, 52–57. [CrossRef]
45. Thomas, R.J.; Kottke, T.E.; Brekke, M.J.; Brekke, L.N.; Brandel, C.L.; Aase, L.A.; DeBoer, S.W. Attempts at changing dietary and exercise habits to reduce risk of cardiovascular disease: Who's doing what in the community? *Prev. Cardiol.* **2002**, *5*, 102–108. [CrossRef]
46. Sallis, J.F.; Cervero, R.B.; Ascher, W.; Henderson, K.A.; Kraft, M.K.; Kerr, J. An ecological approach to creating active living communities. *Annu. Rev. Public Health* **2006**, *27*, 297–322. [CrossRef]
47. Muehlbauer, T.; Roth, R.; Bopp, M.; Granacher, U. An exercise sequence for progression in balance training. *J. Strength Cond. Res.* **2012**, *26*, 568–574. [CrossRef] [PubMed]
48. McLeroy, K.R.; Bibeau, D.; Steckler, A.; Glanz, K. An ecological perspective on health promotion programs. *Health Educ. Q.* **1988**, *15*, 351–377. [CrossRef] [PubMed]
49. Schmidt, L.L.; Johnson, S.; Genoe, M.R.; Jeffery, B.; Crawford, J. Social Interaction and Physical Activity among Rural Older Adults: A Scoping Review. *J. Aging Phys. Act.* **2022**, *30*, 495–509. [CrossRef] [PubMed]
50. Higgins, E.T. Value from regulatory fit. *Curr. Dir. Psychol. Sci.* **2005**, *14*, 209–213. [CrossRef]
51. Newall, N.E.; Menec, V.H. Loneliness and social isolation of older adults: Why it is important to examine these social aspects together. *J. Soc. Pers. Relatsh.* **2019**, *36*, 925–939. [CrossRef]
52. Schrempft, S.; Jackowska, M.; Hamer, M.; Steptoe, A. Associations between social isolation, loneliness, and objective physical activity in older men and women. *BMC Public Health* **2019**, *19*, 74. [CrossRef]
53. Sebastião, E.; Mirda, D. Group-based physical activity as a means to reduce social isolation and loneliness among older adults. *Aging Clin. Exp. Res.* **2021**, *33*, 2003–2006. [CrossRef]
54. Li, G.; Li, X.; Chen, L. Personally tailored exercises for improving physical outcomes for older adults in the community: A systematic review. *Arch. Gerontol. Geriatr.* **2022**, *101*, 104707. [CrossRef]
55. Cederbom, S.; Arkkukangas, M. Impact of the fall prevention Otago Exercise Programme on pain among community-dwelling older adults: A short-and long-term follow-up study. *Clin. Interv. Aging* **2019**, *14*, 721. [CrossRef]
56. Peeters, G.; van Schoor, N.M.; Cooper, R.; Tooth, L.; Kenny, R.A. Should prevention of falls start earlier? Co-ordinated analyses of harmonised data on falls in middle-aged adults across four population-based cohort studies. *PLoS ONE* **2018**, *13*, e0201989.
57. Musich, S.; Wang, S.S.; Hawkins, K.; Greame, C. The frequency and health benefits of physical activity for older adults. *Popul. Health Manag.* **2017**, *20*, 199–207. [CrossRef] [PubMed]
58. Penzer, F.; Duchateau, J.; Baudry, S. Effects of short-term training combining strength and balance exercises on maximal strength and upright standing steadiness in elderly adults. *Exp. Gerontol.* **2015**, *61*, 38–46. [CrossRef] [PubMed]
59. Hu, M.H.; Woollacott, M.H. Multisensory training of standing balance in older adults: I. Postural stability and one-leg stance balance. *J. Gerontol.* **1994**, *49*, M52–M61. [CrossRef] [PubMed]

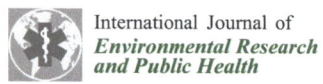

Article

The Role of Physical Function in the Association between Physical Activity and Gait Speed in Older Adults: A Mediation Analysis

Marcelo de Maio Nascimento [1,*], Élvio Rúbio Gouveia [2,3,4], Adilson Marques [5,6], Bruna R. Gouveia [3,4,7,8], Priscila Marconcin [5,9], Cíntia França [2,3] and Andreas Ihle [4,10,11]

1. Department of Physical Education, Federal University of Vale do São Francisco, Petrolina 56304-917, Brazil
2. Department of Physical Education and Sport, University of Madeira, 9020-105 Funchal, Portugal
3. Laboratory for Robotics and Engineering System (LARSYS), Interactive Technologies Institute, 9020-105 Funchal, Portugal
4. Center for the Interdisciplinary Study of Gerontology and Vulnerability, University of Geneva, 1205 Geneva, Switzerland
5. Interdisciplinary Centre for the Study of Human Performance (CIPER), Faculty of Human Kinetics, University of Lisbon, 1495-751 Lisbon, Portugal
6. Instituto de Saúde Ambiental (ISAMB), Faculty of Medicine, University of Lisbon, 1649-020 Lisbon, Portugal
7. Regional Directorate of Health, Secretary of Health of the Autonomous Region of Madeira, 9004-515 Funchal, Portugal
8. Saint Joseph of Cluny Higher School of Nursing, 9050-535 Funchal, Portugal
9. KinesioLab, Research Unit in Human Movement Analysis, Piaget Institute, 2805-059 Almada, Portugal
10. Department of Psychology, University of Geneva, 1205 Geneva, Switzerland
11. Swiss National Centre of Competence in Research LIVES–Overcoming Vulnerability: Life Course Perspectives, 1015 Lausanne, Switzerland
* Correspondence: marcelo.nascimento@univasf.edu.br; Tel.: +55-(87)-21016856

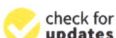

Citation: Nascimento, M.d.M.; Gouveia, É.R.; Marques, A.; Gouveia, B.R.; Marconcin, P.; França, C.; Ihle, A. The Role of Physical Function in the Association between Physical Activity and Gait Speed in Older Adults: A Mediation Analysis. *Int. J. Environ. Res. Public Health* **2022**, *19*, 12581. https://doi.org/10.3390/ijerph191912581

Academic Editors: Andy Pringle and Nicola Kime

Received: 12 July 2022
Accepted: 18 August 2022
Published: 1 October 2022

Publisher's Note: MDPI stays neutral with regard to jurisdictional claims in published maps and institutional affiliations.

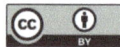

Copyright: © 2022 by the authors. Licensee MDPI, Basel, Switzerland. This article is an open access article distributed under the terms and conditions of the Creative Commons Attribution (CC BY) license (https://creativecommons.org/licenses/by/4.0/).

Simple Summary: Aging is associated with vulnerability in terms of a natural decline of most physiological systems, and, consequently, physical function (PF) performance (e.g., cardiorespiratory performance, muscle strength, flexibility, speed, balance) decreases. Adequate physical activity (PA) levels are essential to maintaining or increasing PF performance, directly influencing gait speed (GS). Having a fast GS increases the older adult's capacity to perform daily tasks safely and remain autonomous at an advanced age. Our study aimed to explore the mediating role of PF in the relationship between PA and GS in a large sample of older adults from the north of Brazil. Regarding the PA-total level, the analysis showed that a fast GS was partially mediated by approximately 19% by a better PF performance. PF partially mediated the association between PA-sport and GS in approximately 9%, and PF partially mediated the association between PA-leisure and GS in 46%. We observed a significant and negative association between PA-housework and GS. Thus, PF partially mediated the association in about 9% of cases. Consequently, our study suggests that among older adults, PF plays a crucial role in mediating the association between PA and GS levels in the vulnerable aging population.

Abstract: Adequate levels of physical function (PF) are essential for vulnerable older adults to perform their daily tasks safely and remain autonomous. Our objective was to explore the mediating role of PF in the relationship between physical activity (PA) and gait speed (GS) in a large sample of older adults from the north of Brazil. This is a cross-sectional study that analyzed 697 older adults (mean age 70.35 ± 6.86 years) who participated in the project "Health, Lifestyle, and Physical Fitness in Older Adults in Amazonas" (SEVAAI). PA was assessed using the Baecke Questionnaire, PF using the Senior Fitness Test, and GS using the 50-foot Walk Test. Mediation pathways were analyzed to test the possible mediating role of PF between specific PA domains (PA-total score, PA-housework, PA-sport, PA-leisure) and GS. Regarding PA-total, the analysis showed that high-performance GS was partially mediated in approximately 19% by better PF performance. Moreover, the PF could partially mediate the association between PA-sport and PA-leisure with GS, at levels of approximately 9% and 46%, respectively. An inverse relationship was observed between PA-housework (sedentary lifestyle) and GS. This association was partially mediated to an extent of approximately 9% by better PF performance. We conclude that PF plays a crucial role in mediating the association between PA and GS among vulnerable older adults.

Keywords: aging; sedentary behavior; physical activity; physical function; mobility; vulnerability; older adults

1. Introduction

Physical function (PF) is strongly related to the human ability to perform activities related to daily living [1,2]. Especially in old age, adequate levels of PF are essential for physical and motor independence, which are necessary for an autonomous life [3]. With vulnerability, PF can decrease dramatically [4]. The most common manifestation of poor health status among the older population is represented by the loss of functioning [5]. Therefore, being an older person and having an impaired PF (e.g., with respect to cardiorespiratory performance, muscle strength, flexibility, speed, or balance) decreases the chance of having a good health condition, quality of life, and well-being [6]. Moreover, having a low level of physical function (PF), and pursuing sedentary behavior (SB) [7], which may be common in the older population [8], contributes to the individual having a low level of PA [9]. Thus, the combination of a low level of PF with a sedentary lifestyle impairs the mobility of older adults.

Mobility is defined as the human ability to move independently and safely in the environment [10]. In old age, mobility problems, including changes in gait speed (GS), are considered early indicators of physical health decline, a warning sign of functional disability [11]. Changes in mobility can negatively affect an older person's autonomy [12], compromising their quality of life and well-being [13]. A low GS may result from endogenous changes caused by physiological aging, such as the loss of muscle strength, central/peripheral nervous systems, and proprioceptive feedback [14,15]. GS impairment is also strongly associated with a greater chance of falling [16]. Among older adults, falls represent a considerable risk to health and quality of life, and are responsible for injuries, days of hospitalization, and enhanced functional incapacity [17,18].

Concerning PA, its performance is classified into levels of intensity, including low intensity (e.g., daily activities such as cooking, cleaning, and working in the garden), moderate intensity and high intensity (e.g., physical exercise) [19]. Regardless of age group, having a low PA level represents an increased risk of developing chronic diseases [20] and a decreased chance of maintaining an autonomous life. Moreover, previous studies have associated low levels of PA with gait disturbances [17,19]. A useful strategy for combating low PA, which potentiates SB, is to increase PF levels [20,21]. In practice, this can be achieved through the regular performance of exercises focused on muscle strength, power, flexibility, cardiorespiratory endurance, postural control, and activities designed to enhance mobility [10,21].

The relationship between gait performance and age is inversely proportional [22]. Thus, the spatial and spatio-temporal parameters of gait tend to decrease [23]. Therefore, when aging is accompanied by low levels of PA and PF becomes insufficient, the performance of the GS automatically declines [24,25]. For this reason, comparatively sedentary older adults adopt a more cautious walking style than active ones, taking shorter and slower steps [26]. Therefore, in situations that require an increase in GS, older adults tend to increase cadence rather than stride length, while younger individuals do the opposite [27].

The relationships between aging, PA, PF, and gait parameters have been extensively studied [20,28,29]. However, the causes of the decrease in GS and changes in other gait patterns (e.g., cadence, stride time, step time, single support, double support, foot off, stride length, step length, time of stance, swing) are not entirely clear [7,30,31]. Furthermore, it is also unclear what weight each specific domain involved in the objective assessment of

PA (e.g., PA-housework, PA-sport, PA-leisure) exerts on the GS of the cognitively normal and healthy older population. Thus, it is important to develop studies that expand our understanding of this relationship, and the findings may favor the creation of public health policy targets for specific domains of PA. Another critical point in the relationship between PA, PF, and GS, is better understanding the mechanisms of these variables in older adults residing in a given geographic area. In healthcare, geographic information plays an essential role in disease surveillance, management and analysis [32]. To the best of our knowledge, no study has addressed the mediating role of PF in the relationship between total PA and GS in the older population of Northern Brazil. Compared to other Brazilian states, the inhabitants of this region still live in conditions of extreme socioeconomic vulnerability [33,34]. According to the Brazilian Society of Geriatrics and Gerontology [35], this negatively affects the aging process of these citizens.

Thus, knowing that moderate to high levels of PF can improve GS performance [16,35], that there is a positive and direct relationship between PA and PF [24,36,37], and that high PF levels are essential to improving and/or maintaining adequate levels of GS [6,38], this study aimed to explore the mediating role of PF in the relationship between PA and GS in a large sample of older adults.

2. Materials and Methods

2.1. Study Design

This is an analytical cross-sectional observational study carried out in the Amazonas state, Northern Brazil. Participants took part in a research project entitled "Health, Lifestyle and Fitness in Adults and Elderly in Amazonas" (SEVAAI), carried out between 2016 and 2017. Participants were recruited through newspapers, churches, support centers, groups, or associations of older people in the municipalities of Manaus, Fonte Boa, and Apuí. The procedures followed the ethical principles, contained in Resolution 466/12 of the National Health Council of the Ministry of Health, evaluated and approved by the Human Research Ethics Committee of the University of the State of Amazonas (n° 1,599,258–CAAE: 56519616.0000.5016).

2.2. Sample Size

For the sample size calculation, we used the G*Power [39]. A priori, using the F family tests, linear regression analysis, with two tested predictors from a total number of 5, indicated that to detect a small relation of $r = 0.04$, with a two-tailed alpha probability of 0.01 and a power of 0.99, the sample would need to comprise at minimum 691 individuals.

2.3. Participants and Eligibility

The inclusion criteria adopted were: (1) living in one of the three cities in Manaus mentioned above; (2) minimum age of 60 years; (3) able to walk independently and perform physical assessments; (4) present autonomy and independence to carry out activities of daily living; (5) no indication of serious health problems (medical contraindications for the practice of physical activity). An exclusion criterion was adopted: score < 15/30 on the Mini-Mental State Examination (MMSE) [40]. This criterion was considered the limit of inability to understand and follow the SEVAAI study protocol. All participants were informed about the investigation procedures and voluntarily signed an informed consent form. In the SEVAAI study, 701 people met the criteria and were included.

Figure 1 shows the flowchart with the study sample selection. In our mediation study, four participants from the original SEVAAI study database were excluded, one due to Parkinson's disease ($n = 1$), and three due to Alzheimer's disease ($n = 3$). Thus, the final sample consisted of 697 participants, totaling 267 men (71.4 ± 7.0 years) and 430 women (69.7 ± 6.6 years).

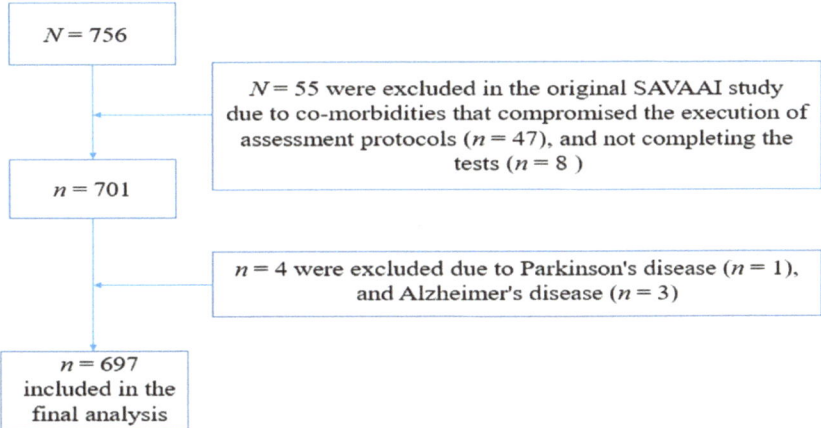

Figure 1. Flowchart of study sample.

2.4. Data Collection

2.4.1. Demographics and Clinical Data

The collection of information on gender, age, years of education, falls, medication, visual and hearing impairment, and blood pressure was obtained through self-report, obtained individually through face-to-face interviews using health questionnaire employed in the "FallProof!" Program [41]. The procedure was conducted by specially trained field team members.

2.4.2. Anthropometry

Body mass index (BMI) was measured using an anthropometric scale and a Welmy® stadiometer coupled with 0.1 cm and 0.1 kg [42], and calculated from weight and height (kg/m^2).

2.4.3. Cognitive Function

Mini-Mental State Examination (MMSE) was used to detect possible cases of dementia [43]. In the original SEVAAI study, a score of <15/30 points was assumed to be the disability threshold for participants to understand the protocols and follow all assessments.

2.4.4. Physical Activity

The level of physical activity (PA) was measured using the Brazilian version of the Baecke Questionnaire for older adults [44], adapted from the original questionnaire by Voorrips et al. [45]. This instrument is divided into three sections based on lifestyle habits for the last 12 months: (1) household activities (PA-housework); (2) sports activities (PA-sport), only regular activities lasting at least one hour per week; and (3) free time activities (PA-leisure). In this study, the following scores were used: specific physical activity domains (PA-housework, PA-sport, PA-leisure), and the total score (PA-total), calculated from the mean scores of the three domains.

2.4.5. Physical Function

PF was evaluated using the Senior Fitness Test (STF) [46]. For the present study, six physical function components were selected as physical fitness parameters: (1) lower body strength (quadriceps, glutes): after a signal, participants were asked to get up from a chair and then return to a fully seated position, repeating the task as many times as possible for 30 sec; (2) arm curl, to assess upper-body strength: after the signal, participants were instructed to flex and extend the elbow of the dominant hand, throughout the range of motion, lifting a weight (2.3 kg dumbbell for women, and 3.6 kg dumbbell for men) as many times as possible for 30 sec. The score was determined by the total number of repetitions performed in 30 sec; (3) flexibility in the lower body (sit-and-reach chair/cm): participants were asked to sit on the edge of a chair, with one leg bent and the other extended straight in front, keeping the heel on the floor, without bending the knee. In this position, the participants extended their hands in front of them, slowly sliding over the extended leg towards the feet. The score was the number of centimeters before the toes (lowest score) or reached beyond the toes (highest score); (4) flexibility in the upper body (back scratch/cm): participants placed one hand behind the same lateral shoulder with the forearm pronated, fingers extended, the other hand behind the back, fingers extended. The score was determined by the centimeters left for the middle fingers to touch those of the other hand (lower score), or centimeters overlapping each other (higher score); (5) agility/dynamic balance (8-foot up-and-go/s): participants were fully seated in a chair, hands on thighs and feet flat on the floor. After a signal, they got up from the chair, walked as quickly as possible (without running) around a cone placed 8 ft (2.44 m) in front of the chair, returning and sitting fully in the chair. The result was established by the time in seconds required to rise from a sitting position, walk and return to a sitting position; and (6) aerobic endurance (6-min walk test/m): after a signal, participants walked as fast as possible (without running) along a marked path, as many times as possible. The score was determined by the distance (meters) covered in the six-minute interval. A sum of the scores for all indicators provided by the SFT was used to calculate a continuous overall measure of the participants' physical function (PF total = CST + ACT + CSAR + BST + FUG + MWT6).

2.4.6. Gait

GS was assessed using the 30-Foot (9 m) Walk Test [41]. Participants were required to walk at their preferred speed. For each participant, three measurements were collected, and the best performance was considered in the analysis. A full description of the test administration instructions for the test is reported in Rose [41].

2.4.7. Statistical Analysis

The main characteristics of the participants (i.e., sociodemographic, clinical, blood pressure, BMI and MMSE) are presented using descriptive statistics. These data are presented on the basis of the total number of individuals, and although our study does not focus on drawing group comparisons, these data are also presented in two groups according to the total score of the Baecke Questionnaire [44]. The calculation was performed based on the mean of the PA-total: PA-total < 2.57 points (low level), and PA-total $\geq$ 2.57 points (high level). From this, the main characteristics of the participants were compared using the Chi-square test (categorical variables) and the parametric Student's t test for independent samples (continuous variables). In the descriptive statistics, only sociodemographic, clinical, blood pressure, BMI, and MMSE variables were included. Prior to the mediation analysis (the main objective of the investigation), the strength and direction of the association between the study variables (PA-total, PA-housework, PA-sport, PA-leisure, PF, and GS) were verified. The examination was performed by bivariate analyses, and the results were presented by Pearson's correlation coefficients (r), considering the following interpretation: 0.1 = small, 0.3 = medium, and $\geq$0.5 = large [47].

Finally, we used the statistical mediation analysis method (Figure 2), making it possible to expand and qualify the understanding of how physical activity acts on GS influenced by the indirect effect of PF. A complete mediation would be observed if, with the inclusion of objectively measured PF (mediator variable), the size of association between the independent variable (PA-total, PA-housework, PA-sport, PA-leisure) and the dependent variable (GS) became non-significant, indicated by its confidence interval including zero [48]. A partial mediation would occur if the observed relationship between independent variable and dependent variable became weaker after the inclusion of objectively measured PF (mediator variable).

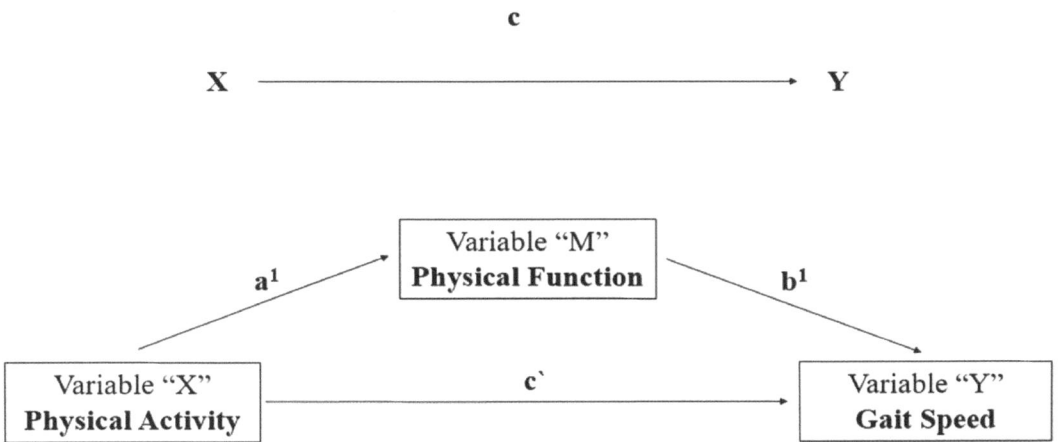

Figure 2. Linear mediation relationships to examine the mediating role of PF in the relationship between PA and GS. Path (a) = association between PA-Activity (X) with mediator (M) Physical Function (Y), Path (b) = association between mediator (M) Physical Function with Gait Speed (Y), Path c′ = direct effect (X-Y).

The effects represented by the regression coefficients in Equations (1) and (2) were estimated with a computational complement to the SPSS program using PROCESS v4.0: an analysis of model estimation developed by Hayes [49]. The coefficients a1 and b1 described in the equation (Figure 2) were calculated using least squares regression, as follows:

$$M = a_0 + a_1 X + r \quad (1)$$

$$M = b_0 + c' X + b_1 M + r \quad (2)$$

The mediation hypothesis test was estimated using a confidence interval (95%) with bias correction and acceleration (BCa) by the Bootstrapping method with bias correction (5000 re-samplings). Thus, the indirect effect was considered significant when the confidence interval did not include zero [48]. The calculation of the proportion of the mediation effect was obtained as follows: subtraction 1 minus the result of the division between the direct effect and the total effect [49]. Furthermore, the results illustrated in the figures correspond to standardized parameters β.

3. Results

3.1. Main Characteristics of the Participants

The mean age of the group with low PA was 71.17 ± 7.28 years, while participants with high PA indicated a mean of 69.53 ± 6.31 years (Table 1). Regarding PA, except for the PA-housework domain ($p = 0.024$), the group with high PA exhibited better scores in the PA-sport and PA-leisure domains ($p < 0.001$). The high PA group members indicated better performance on functional tests, except for the 30 s chair stand test (CST) ($p = 0.790$). Regarding the GS test, members of the low PA group had a lower result than those of the high PA group ($p < 0.001$).

Regarding the descriptive analyses, Table 2 shows the levels of correlation between PA, PF and GS. A positive and small association was found between PA-housework and PA-sport ($r = 0.245$). A negative and small association was found between PA-housework and PA-leisure ($r = -0.005$). PA-leisure was not related to PA-housework. Higher scores on the PA-total were positively and weakly associated with higher scores on the PA-housework ($r = 0.003$), positively and at a medium level with the PA-sport ($r = 0.476$), in addition positively and at a large level with the PA-sport ($r = 0.476$), and PA-leisure ($r = 0.870$). A high level of performance in PA-total was negatively and weakly associated with PA-housework ($r = -0.118$), positively and weakly with PA-sport ($r = 0.139$), and with PA-leisure ($r = 0.160$). High values of GS were negatively and weakly associated with PA-housework ($r = -0.215$), positively and at a medium level with PA-sport ($r = 0.515$), positively and weakly with PA-leisure ($r = 0.075$), and with PA-total ($r = 0.298$). Finally, high performance in the GS indicated a positive and medium association with higher scores in the performance of PA-total ($r = 0.302$).

Table 1. Main characteristics of participants, according to the level of physical activity.

Variable	Low PA Mean (SD)	High PA Mean (SD)	Total Mean (SD)	p-Value
	(n = 348)	(n = 349)	(n = 697)	
Age (years)	71.17 ± 7.28	69.53 ± 6.31	70.35 ± 6.36	0.007
Sex (n) (%)				
women	196 (56.3)	234 (67.0)	430 (61.7)	0.004
men	152 (43.7)	115 (33.0)	267 (38.3)	
BMI (k/m^2)	27.88 ± 5.00	25.30 ± 3.86	28.21 ± 4.93	0.059
Education (years)	3.65 ± 4.72	7.03 ± 7.80	5.35 ± 5.55	<0.001
MMSE (n)	23.50 ± 4.40	25.30 ± 3.86	24.41 ± 4.23	<0.001
Falls n (%)	121 (34.8)	106 (30.4)	227 (32.6)	0.216
Medication (n)	1.83 ± 1.83	1.95 ± 1.74	1.89 ± 1.79	0.255
Comorbidities (n) (%)				
Hypertension	201 (57.8)	194 (55.6)	395 (56.7)	0.563
Visual impairment	289 (83.0)	293 (84.0)	582 (83.5)	0.012
Hearing problems	85 (24.4)	95 (27.2)	180 (25.8)	0.555
Physical activity				
PA-housework (n)	2.87 ± 0.44	2.78 ± 0.45	2.82 ± 0.47	0.024
PA-sport (n)	2.00 ± 0.40	2.35 ± 0.62	2.18 ± 0.55	<0.001
PA-leisure (n)	2.70 ± 0.51	2.93 ± 0.55	2.71 ± 0.54	<0.001
PA-total (n)	2.52 ± 0.45	2.68 ± 1.53	2.57 ± 0.52	<0.001
Physical function				
CST (n)	11.71 ± 3.41	11.74 ± 3.02	11.73 ± 3.22	0.790
ACT (n)	13.92 ± 4.41	12.36 ± 3.91	13.14 ± 4.24	<0.001
CSAR (cm)	1.97 ± 8.02	3.77 ± 10.70	2.87 ± 9.50	0.021
BST (cm)	−12.80 ± 12.90	−6.87 ± 10.61	−9.84 ± 12.17	<0.001
FUG (seg.)	6.71 ± 2.45	5.88 ± 1.20	6.30 ± 1.98	<0.001
MWT 6 (m)	400.47 ± 89.90	438.98 ± 80.16	419.75 ± 87.25	<0.001
PF total (score)	422.75 ± 94.84	465.86 ± 86.11	444.40 ± 93.04	<0.001
Gait speed (m/s)	1.17 ± 0.36	1.52 ± 0.49	1.35 ± 0.46	<0.001

BMI: body mass index; MMSE: Mini Mental State Examination; CST: 30 s chair stand test; ACT: 30 s arm curl test; CSAR: chair sit-and-reach test; BST: back scratch test; FUG: foot up-and go test; MWT6: 6-min walk test; $p < 0.05$; CI, confidence interval.

3.2. Mediation Analysis: PF in the Relationship between PA-Total and GS

Regarding the main objective of our study, Figure 3 presents the mediation model used to determine whether PF performance can mediate the effect of PA-total level on GS. The direct effect estimated by the model ($x \to y$) showed a significant positive relationship between the highest level of PA-total and the highest GS, $\beta = 0.03$; 95% CI (0.021–0.039), $t = 6.64$, $p = 0.001$. Path (a) = association between PA-total (x) with mediator Physical Function (m), Path (b) = association between mediator Physical Function (m) with Gait Speed (y), The total effect of the model ($x \rightarrow y$) indicated a significant positive relationship between a high PA-total and high GS performance, $\beta = 0.04$; 95% CI (0.028–0.047), $t = 8.14$, $p = 0.001$, and a significant positive indirect effect was indicated between high PA-total and high GS performance, $\beta = 0.01$ (95% CI BCa = 0.0347–0.010). Thus, the proportion of the total effect of FA-total on GS mediated by PF was approximately 16%.

Table 2. Associations between analyzed variables.

Variable	PA-Housework	PA-Sport	PA-Leisure	PA-Total	PF
PA-sport	0.245 ***				
PA-leisure	−0.005 ns	0.000 ns			
PA-total	0.003 ns	0.476 ***	0.870 ***		
PF	0.118 **	0.139 ***	0.160 ***	0.226 ***	
Gait speed	−0.215 ***	0.515 ***	0.075 *	0.298 ***	0.302 ***

PA = physical activity; PF = physical function; * $p < 0.05$; ** $p < 0.01$; *** $p < 0.001$; ns = non-significant, $p > 0.05$.

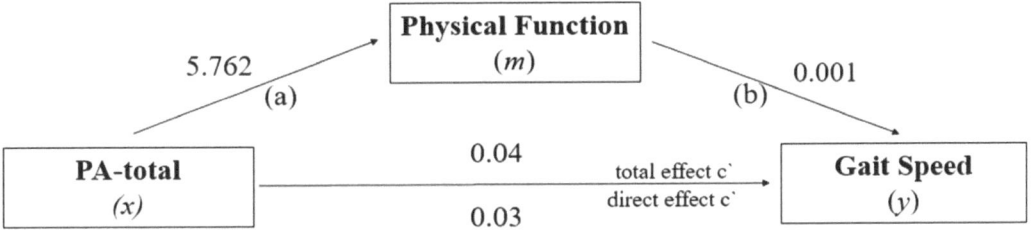

Figure 3. PF model as a mediator of the effect of PA-total on GS.

3.3. Mediation Analysis: PF in the Relationship between PA-Housework and GS

Figure 4 presents the estimate for the PA-housework specific domain. The direct effect estimated by the model ($x \rightarrow y$) indicated a significant negative relationship between the highest level of PA-housework with low GS performance, $\beta = -0.25$; 95% CI (−0.3185–0.1847), $t = -7.38$, $p = 0.000$. Path (a) = association between PA-housework (x) with mediator Physical Function (m), Path (b) = association between mediator Physical Function (m) with Gait Speed (y). The total effect of the model ($x \rightarrow y$) also showed a significant negative relationship between PA-housework and GS, $\beta = -0.21$; 95% CI (−0.2841–0.1430), $t = -5.94$, $p = 0.001$. In view of the indirect effect, a significant negative association was found between high PA-housework and low GS performance, $\beta = -0.04$ (95% CI BCa = 0.0127–0.0653). Thus, the proportion of the total effect of PA-housework on GS mediated by PF was approximately 9%.

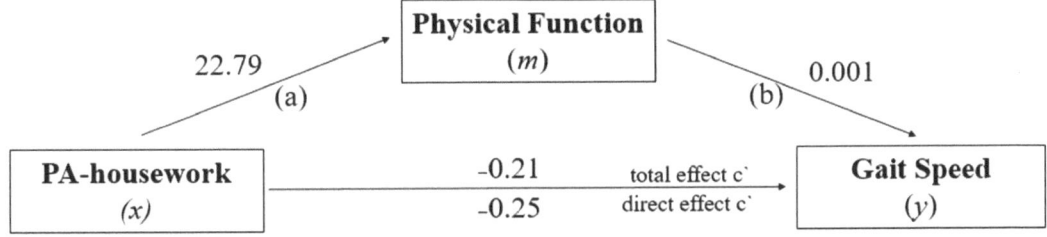

Figure 4. PF model as a mediator of the effect of PA-housework on GS.

3.4. Mediation Analysis: PF in the Relationship between PA-Sport and GS

In relation to the PA-sport specific domain (Figure 5), the direct effect estimated by the model ($x \rightarrow y$) revealed a non-significant relationship between the highest level of PA-sport and the highest performance of GS, $\beta = 0.12$; 95% CI (0.1370–0.4816), $t = -15.19$, $p = 0.132$. Path (a) = association between PA-sport (x) with mediator Physical Function (m), Path (b) = association between mediator Physical Function (m) with Gait Speed (y), The total effect of the model ($x \rightarrow y$) also showed a non-significant relationship between PA-sport and GS, $\beta = 0.13$; 95% CI (-0.1457–0.5142), $t = 15.78$, $p = 0.086$. On the other hand, the indirect effect indicated a significant positive association between high PA-sport and high GS performance, $\beta = 0.01$ (95% CI BCa = 0.0039–0.0133). Thus, the proportion of the total effect of PA-sport on GS mediated by PF was approximately 9%.

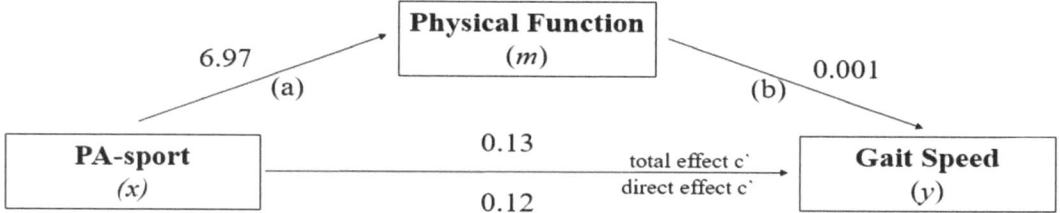

Figure 5. PF model as a mediator of the effect of PA-sport on GS.

3.5. Mediation Analysis: PF in the Relationship between PA-Leisure and GS

For the PA-leisure specific domain (Figure 6), the direct effect estimated by the model ($x \rightarrow y$) revealed a non-significant direct relationship between the highest level of PA-leisure and the highest GS, $\beta = 0.04$; 95% CI (0.0143–0.0249), $t = 0.67$, $p = 0.496$. Path (a) = association between PA-leisure (x) with mediator Physical Function (m), Path (b) = association between mediator Physical Function (m) with Gait Speed (y), The total effect of the model ($x \rightarrow y$) also showed a positive and non-significant relationship between high PA-leisure and high GS performance, $\beta = 0.02$; 95% CI (-0.1457–0.5142), $t = 1.91$, $p = 0.055$. The indirect effect showed a positive significant relationship between high PA-leisure and high GS performance, $\beta = 0.08$ (95% CI BCa = 0.0037–0.0111). Thus, the proportion of the total effect of PA-leisure on PF-mediated GS was approximately 46%.

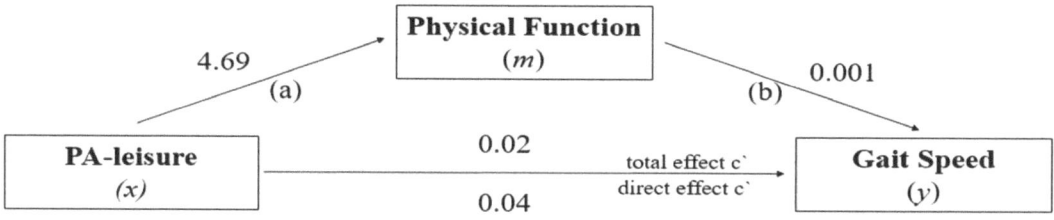

Figure 6. PF model as a mediator of the effect of PA-leisure on GS.

4. Discussion

This study aimed to explore the mediating role of PF in the relationship between PA-total and their specific domains with GS. Our findings showed that high levels of PA-total, PA-sport and PA-leisure were positively associated with better GS performance. In relation to total-PA, the analysis showed that a high GS was partially mediated by approximately 19% by better PF performance. Second, in relation to PA-sport, when PF was placed as a mediator, the direct and total effects of the path between x-y became non-significant. This means that PF partially mediated the association between PA-sport and GS in approximately 9%. Third, the inclusion of PF as a mediator showed that the direct and total pathway effects between PA-leisure and GS were not significant. This means that PF could partially mediate the association between PA-leisure and GS in approximately 46%.

The specific domain PA-housework was negatively associated with GS performance. Thus, a high PA-housework score was partially mediated by approximately 9% by better PF performance. The negative effect (direct and total) indicated by PA-housework on GS was mediated by a positive indirect effect of PF. This result suggests the importance of reducing SB levels in older adults and increasing their PF levels through physical exercise. In this way, it is possible to attenuate negative associations between PA and GS and, consequently, improve mobility, functionality, and quality of life [16]. SB is considered the main risk factor for noncommunicable diseases [50], responsible each year for the death of 41 million people, equivalent to 71% of all deaths in the world [51]. For this reason, the WHO has suggested guidelines for the older adult population entitled 'Global Recommendations on Physical Activity for Health' [52], as well as the American College of Sports Medicine [53]. The positions posted by both are similar, suggesting a minimum of 150 min of moderate-intensity aerobic activity per week, or at least 75 min of vigorous-intensity aerobic activity, or an equivalent combination. In addition, muscle-strengthening activities should be done on 2 or more days, and people with limited mobility should do balance exercises to prevent falls on 3 or more days. From this perspective, reaching the recommended levels of aerobic fitness, as well as a high physical condition can benefit the older adult population to improve several aspects associated with a good quality of life [54].

Age has an inversely proportional effect on PF [55]. Thus, an increase in PA levels may consequently generate an improvement in PF, presumably benefiting variables associated with mobility such as muscle strength, balance, and cardiovascular endurance [56], and notwithstanding, the GS itself [21]. Among sexagenarians, the annual muscle loss varies from 1 to 2%, reaching 3.4% after age 75 [4]. Furthermore, the loss of muscle strength is different between the sexes and between the lower and upper limbs. On the other hand, it is known that physiological changes resulting from aging, as well as functional limitations associated with mobility, can be mitigated or prevented through physical exercise, increasing daily/weekly PF levels [20].

Our evidence that a higher level of PF is associated with a higher GS is in accordance with previous investigations. In a cross-sectional study (n = 1352; 68.6 ± 7.5 years), the association of PA-total with GS was observed for those aged ≥ 75 years [57]. Therefore, moderate and vigorous PA levels were related to lower-body physical performance (GS and the task of rising from a chair) and handgrip strength. Regarding sedentary time, the authors identified inverse associations with lower-body physical performance [57], which can negatively affect GS. This result is in agreement with our finding that the performance of the GS tends to be slower, when the level of PA-housework was also low.

At advanced age, the interdependence between PA, PF, and GS is considerable and decisive for the individual's autonomy. High levels of PA [58,59] and high GS performance are essential for safely performing instrumental activities of daily living [60]. A GS performance of 1 m/s is considered the ideal minimum threshold for an older adult to have a more stable gait pattern [23]. Gait is also a strong indicator of health and quality of life [10]. On the other hand, a low GS may be associated with poor cognitive performance [61], as well as leg muscle weakness [62], and consequently, these factors together may increase the risk of falls [60,63,64]. Moreover, slow GS values can also be indicative of future cognitive impairment [65]. For this reason, GS plays a role as a marker of cognitive decline. A longitudinal study indicated a negative relationship between PA and cognitive decline during vulnerable aging [66]. For this reason, a suggested strategy to reverse/mitigate this relationship is to promote PA levels. Consequently, there is a greater chance that cognitive functions will remain adequate [67]. Another population-based longitudinal investigation revealed an increased risk of morbidity [68], and mortality for older adults who showed a rapid decline in GS [69,70]. In a population-based cohort study conducted with older adult Brazilians (>60 years; n = 332) to assess the relationship between PA and SB with mortality revealed SB as a potential risk for mortality [71]. Moreover, the analysis pointed to SB as a barrier for older adults to present moderate to vigorous PA levels.

It is worth noting that PA and/or SB levels may be strongly associated with socioeconomic factors. In a cross-sectional study that used data from a national household-based survey carried out by the Brazilian Ministry of Health (n = 60,202) to examine the population's health status, lifestyle, and chronic diseases [72], no differences were found regarding gender. Still, differences were found in ethnicity (being older adult black or white), weekly practice of physical exercise, income, and years of education. Having a low income and few years of education can prevent older adults from practicing physical exercises, as well as demonstrate low involvement in leisure activities. In another population-based study in in southeast Brazil (n = 621; 70.8 ± 8.1 years), the prevalence of SB was 70.1% [73]. Moreover, being male and over 80 years, having few years of education, low functional capacity, smoking, and not having private health insurance were associated with SB. Although it was not our objective, we partially corroborate these results. Indeed, in our study, members of the high PA group indicated 3.38 (48%) more years of education than those in the low PA group.

The present study's findings confirmed the outcomes of previous studies, suggesting that high levels of PA are essential for promoting and/or preventing the decline of functions involved in PF, which plays a key role in healthy aging [74], including preserved GS. The ability to walk depends on the good function and interaction of a set of systems (e.g., musculoskeletal, visual, central, and peripheral nervous) and cardiorespiratory fitness [68]. Highlighting the role of gait quality in the life of the older adults, it can be said that small changes in GS (an increase of 0.1 m/s) were related to an increase in the predicted survival of 10 years, with a variation of 19% to 87% for men, and 35% to 91% for women [68]. In this context, we reiterate that to reduce or prevent loss of speed during gait, it is essential to increase moderate/vigorous PA frequency and duration throughout the week [75].

The cross-sectional design used in this study is a limitation, since it does not allow conclusions about the cause-and-effect relationship between PA and GS when mediated by the role of PF Moreover, cross-sectional data cannot support causal inferences, but mediation analysis is considered a robust approach, therefore making it possible to infer potential causalities. A strong point of this investigation is the more in-depth results of the relationship between the three specific domains of PA with GS when mediated by PF. Another strong point is the inclusion of a large representative sample from a defined geographic area [32] (the municipalities of Manaus, Fonte Boa, and Apuí). Thus, this is the first mediation study carried out with community-dwelling older adults from the north of Brazil. The information about PA was self-reported, and therefore, possible bias derived from the data collection must be considered. However, to reduce the risk of bias, the interviews were conducted in person by trained researchers. It is suggested that future investigations focusing on the older population might explore the association between specific domains of PA and GS, investigating the mediating role of PF both in older adults in other regions of Brazil and in other countries to compare and extend our findings. Moreover, we suggest the inclusion of longitudinal monitoring.

5. Conclusions

We conclude that PF is crucial in mediating the association between PA and GS among vulnerable older adults. Our findings also highlight the importance of high levels of PA, particularly PA-sport and PA-leisure, combined with high levels of PF, for older adults' GS to maintain enough mobility to guarantee their autonomy. Therefore, investing in greater engagement of the older population in sports and leisure activities can presumably be an effective, simple, and inexpensive strategy to promote GS, quality of life, and well-being. Finally, this study contributes to a better understanding of the interrelationship between PA, PF, and GS in vulnerable aging, helping to formulate helpful strategies for public health guidance.

Author Contributions: Conceptualization, M.d.M.N., É.R.G. and A.I.; methodology, M.d.M.N. and É.R.G.; software, É.R.G.; validation, M.d.M.N., É.R.G. and B.R.G.; formal analysis, M.d.M.N.; investigation, M.d.M.N., É.R.G., B.R.G. and A.I.; resources, É.R.G., B.R.G. and A.I.; data curation, M.d.M.N. and É.R.G.; writing—original draft preparation, M.d.M.N., É.R.G. and A.I.; writing—review and editing, A.M., C.F., B.R.G. and P.M.; visualization, M.d.M.N. and É.R.G.; supervision, É.R.G., B.R.G. and A.I.; project administration, M.d.M.N., É.R.G. and A.I.; funding acquisition, É.R.G., B.R.G. and A.I. All authors have read and agreed to the published version of the manuscript.

Funding: We acknowledge support from the Swiss National Centre of Competence in Research LIVES–Overcoming vulnerability: life course perspectives, which is funded by the Swiss National Science Foundation (grant number: 51NF40-185901). Moreover, AI acknowledges support from the Swiss National Science Foundation (grant number: 10001C_189407). E.R.G., C.F. and B.R.G. acknowledge support from LARSyS—Portuguese national funding agency for science, research and technology (FCT) pluriannual funding 2020–2023 (Reference: UIDB/50009/2020).

Institutional Review Board Statement: The study was conducted according to the guidelines of the Declaration of Helsinki and had been approved by the local ethics committee before the start of the data collection (ethic committee name: The Research Ethics Committee-Human Beings; approval code: CAAE: 56519616.6.0000.5016, Number: 1.599.258, Brazil Platform; approval date: 20 June 2016).

Informed Consent Statement: Informed consent was obtained from all subjects involved in the study before participation.

Data Availability Statement: The data presented in this study are available upon request from the corresponding author.

Acknowledgments: The authors are grateful to Duarte L. Freitas and Jefferson Jurema for their help in setting up the study as well as Maria A. Tinôco, Floramara T. Machado, Angenay P. Odim, and Bárbara R. Muniz for technical assistance in the data collection and management. We are especially grateful to the older people for their participation and interest.

Conflicts of Interest: The authors declare no conflict of interest. The funders had no role in the design of the study; in the collection, analyses, or interpretation of data; in the writing of the manuscript, or in the decision to publish the results.

References

1. Wang, D.X.M.; Yao, J.; Zirek, Y.; Reijnierse, E.M.; Maier, A.B. Muscle mass, strength, and physical performance predicting activities of daily living: A meta-analysis. *J. Cachexia. Sarcopenia Muscle* **2020**, *11*, 3–25. [CrossRef] [PubMed]
2. Liu, C.; Shiroy, D.M.; Jones, L.Y.; Clark, D.O. Systematic review of functional training on muscle strength, physical functioning, and activities of daily living in older adults. *Eur. Rev. Aging Phys. Act.* **2014**, *11*, 95–106. [CrossRef]
3. Knapik, A.; Brzęk, A.; Famuła-Wąż, A.; Gallert-Kopyto, W.; Szydłak, D.; Marcisz, C.; Plinta, R. The relationship between physical fitness and health self-assessment in elderly. *Medicine* **2019**, *98*, e15984. [CrossRef]
4. Milanović, Z.; Pantelić, S.; Trajković, N.; Sporiš, G.; Kostić, R.; James, N.Z. Age-related decrease in physical activity and functional fitness among elderly men and women. *Clin. Interv. Aging* **2013**, *8*, 549. [CrossRef]
5. Patrizio, E.; Calvani, R.; Marzetti, E.; Cesari, M. Physical functional assessment in older adults. *J. Frailty Aging* **2021**, *10*, 141–149. [CrossRef]
6. McPhee, J.S.; French, D.P.; Jackson, D.; Nazroo, J.; Pendleton, N.; Degens, H. Physical activity in older age: Perspectives for healthy ageing and frailty. *Biogerontology* **2016**, *17*, 567–580. [CrossRef] [PubMed]
7. Kasović, M.; Štefan, L.; Zvonař, M. Domain-Specific and Total Sedentary Behavior Associated with Gait Velocity in Older Adults: The Mediating Role of Physical Fitness. *Int. J. Environ. Res. Public Health* **2020**, *17*, 593. [CrossRef] [PubMed]
8. Lin, Y.-H.; Chen, Y.-C.; Tseng, Y.-C.; Tsai, S.; Tseng, Y.-H. Physical activity and successful aging among middle-aged and older adults: A systematic review and meta-analysis of cohort studies. *Aging* **2020**, *12*, 7704–7716. [CrossRef]
9. Sardinha, L.B.; Santos, D.A.; Silva, A.M.; Baptista, F.; Owen, N. Breaking-up Sedentary Time Is Associated with Physical Function in Older Adults. *J. Gerontol. Ser. A Biol. Sci. Med. Sci.* **2015**, *70*, 119–124. [CrossRef]
10. Ebeling, P.R.; Cicuttini, F.; Scott, D.; Jones, G. Promoting mobility and healthy aging in men: A narrative review. *Osteoporos. Int.* **2019**, *30*, 1911–1922. [CrossRef]
11. Musich, S.; Wang, S.S.; Ruiz, J.; Hawkins, K.; Wicker, E. The impact of mobility limitations on health outcomes among older adults. *Geriatr. Nurs.* **2018**, *39*, 162–169. [CrossRef] [PubMed]
12. Hamacher, D.; Liebl, D.; Hödl, C.; Heßler, V.; Kniewasser, C.K.; Thönnessen, T.; Zech, A. Gait Stability and Its Influencing Factors in Older Adults. *Front. Physiol.* **2019**, *9*, 1955. [CrossRef] [PubMed]

13. van Schooten, K.S.; Pijnappels, M.; Lord, S.R.; van Dieën, J.H. Quality of Daily-Life Gait: Novel Outcome for Trials that Focus on Balance, Mobility, and Falls. *Sensors* **2019**, *19*, 4388. [CrossRef] [PubMed]
14. Aboutorabi, A.; Arazpour, M.; Bahramizadeh, M.; Hutchins, S.W.; Fadayevatan, R. The effect of aging on gait parameters in able-bodied older subjects: A literature review. *Aging Clin. Exp. Res.* **2016**, *28*, 393–405. [CrossRef] [PubMed]
15. Herssens, N.; Verbecque, E.; Hallemans, A.; Vereeck, L.; Van Rompaey, V.; Saeys, W. Do spatiotemporal parameters and gait variability differ across the lifespan of healthy adults? A systematic review. *Gait Posture* **2018**, *64*, 181–190. [CrossRef]
16. Steckhan, G.M.A.; Fleig, L.; Schwarzer, R.; Warner, L.M. Perceived Physical Functioning and Gait Speed as Mediators in the Association Between Fear of Falling and Quality of Life in Old Age. *J. Appl. Gerontol.* **2020**, *41*, 421–429. [CrossRef]
17. Florence, C.S.; Bergen, G.; Atherly, A.; Burns, E.; Stevens, J.; Drake, C. Medical Costs of Fatal and Nonfatal Falls in Older Adults. *J. Am. Geriatr. Soc.* **2018**, *66*, 693–698. [CrossRef]
18. Viswanathan, A.; Sudarsky, L. Balance and gait problems in the elderly. In *Handbook of Clinical Neurology*; Elsevier: Amsterdam, The Netherlands, 2012; Volume 103, pp. 623–634.
19. Carter, S.; Hartman, Y.; Holder, S.; Thijssen, D.H.; Hopkins, N.D. Sedentary Behavior and Cardiovascular Disease Risk: Mediating Mechanisms. *Exerc. Sport Sci. Rev.* **2017**, *45*, 80–86. [CrossRef]
20. Slater, L.; Gilbertson, N.M.; Hyngstrom, A.S. Improving gait efficiency to increase movement and physical activity—The impact of abnormal gait patterns and strategies to correct. *Prog. Cardiovasc. Dis.* **2021**, *64*, 83–87. [CrossRef]
21. Ciprandi, D.; Bertozzi, F.; Zago, M.; Ferreira, C.L.P.; Boari, G.; Sforza, C.; Galvani, C. Study of the association between gait variability and physical activity. *Eur. Rev. Aging Phys. Act.* **2017**, *14*, 19. [CrossRef]
22. Jerome, G.J.; Ko, S.; Kauffman, D.; Studenski, S.A.; Ferrucci, L.; Simonsick, E.M. Gait characteristics associated with walking speed decline in older adults: Results from the Baltimore Longitudinal Study of Aging. *Arch. Gerontol. Geriatr.* **2015**, *60*, 239–243. [CrossRef] [PubMed]
23. Huijben, B.; van Schooten, K.S.; van Dieën, J.H.; Pijnappels, M. The effect of walking speed on quality of gait in older adults. *Gait Posture* **2018**, *65*, 112–116. [CrossRef] [PubMed]
24. Silva, F.M.; Petrica, J.; Serrano, J.; Paulo, R.; Ramalho, A.; Lucas, D.; Ferreira, J.P.; Duarte-Mendes, P. The Sedentary Time and Physical Activity Levels on Physical Fitness in the Elderly: A Comparative Cross Sectional Study. *Int. J. Environ. Res. Public Health* **2019**, *16*, 3697. [CrossRef]
25. Chaabene, H.; Prieske, O.; Herz, M.; Moran, J.; Höhne, J.; Kliegl, R.; Ramirez-Campillo, R.; Behm, D.G.; Hortobágyi, T.; Granacher, U. Home-based exercise programmes improve physical fitness of healthy older adults: A PRISMA-compliant systematic review and meta-analysis with relevance for COVID-19. *Ageing Res. Rev.* **2021**, *67*, 101265. [CrossRef]
26. Cruz-Jimenez, M. Normal Changes in Gait and Mobility Problems in the Elderly. *Phys. Med. Rehabil. Clin. N. Am.* **2017**, *28*, 713–725. [CrossRef] [PubMed]
27. Fukuchi, C.A.; Fukuchi, R.K.; Duarte, M. Effects of walking speed on gait biomechanics in healthy participants: A systematic review and meta-analysis. *Syst. Rev.* **2019**, *8*, 153. [CrossRef]
28. Pau, M.; Leban, B.; Collu, G.; Migliaccio, G.M. Effect of light and vigorous physical activity on balance and gait of older adults. *Arch. Gerontol. Geriatr.* **2014**, *59*, 568–573. [CrossRef]
29. Taraldsen, K.; Helbostad, J.L.; Follestad, T.; Bergh, S.; Selbæk, G.; Saltvedt, I. Gait, physical function, and physical activity in three groups of home-dwelling older adults with different severity of cognitive impairment—A cross-sectional study. *BMC Geriatr.* **2021**, *21*, 670. [CrossRef]
30. Monteiro-Odasso, M.; Schapira, M.; Soriano, E.R.; Varela, M.; Kaplan, R.; Camera, L.A.; Mayorga, L.M. Gait velocity as a single predictor of adverse events in healthy seniors aged 75 years and older. *Gerontol. Soc. Am.* **2005**, *60A*, 1304–1309. [CrossRef]
31. Noce Kirkwood, R.; de Souza Moreira, B.; Mingoti, S.A.; Faria, B.F.; Sampaio, R.F.; Alves Resende, R. The slowing down phenomenon: What is the age of major gait velocity decline? *Maturitas* **2018**, *115*, 31–36. [CrossRef]
32. Fradelos, E.; Papathanasiou, I.; Mitsi, D.; Tsaras, K.; Kleisiaris, C.; Kourkouta, L. Health Based Geographic Information Systems (GIS) and their Applications. *Acta Inform. Medica* **2014**, *22*, 402. [CrossRef]
33. Miranda Goncalves, R.; Moreira Domingos, I. Riverside Population in Amazonas and Inequality in Access to Health. *Rev. Estud. Const. Hermenêutica e Teor. Direito* **2019**, *11*, 99–108.
34. Aracaty, M.L.; de Souza Rojas, S.R. Índice de vulnerabilidade Social vulnerability index (IVS) of the metropolitan regions of Belém do Pará-PA (RMB) and Manaus-AM (RMM). *Econ. Desenv* **2021**, *33*, 1–22.
35. SBGG-Brazilian Society of Geriatrics and Gerontology Mais Idosos Poucos Geriátras [More Older Adult Few Geriatricians]. Available online: http://www.sbgg-sp.com.br/pub/mais-idosos-poucos-geriatras/ (accessed on 26 March 2019).
36. Garcia Meneguci, C.A.; Meneguci, J.; Sasaki, J.E.; Tribess, S.; Júnior, J.S.V. Physical activity, sedentary behavior and functionality in older adults: A cross-sectional path analysis. *PLoS ONE* **2021**, *16*, e0246275. [CrossRef] [PubMed]
37. Yatsugi, H.; Chen, T.; Chen, S.; Liu, X.; Kishimoto, H. The Associations between Objectively Measured Physical Activity and Physical Function in Community-Dwelling Older Japanese Men and Women. *Int. J. Environ. Res. Public Health* **2021**, *19*, 369. [CrossRef] [PubMed]
38. Cunningham, C.; O' Sullivan, R.; Caserotti, P.; Tully, M.A. Consequences of physical inactivity in older adults: A systematic review of reviews and meta-analyses. *Scand. J. Med. Sci. Sports* **2020**, *30*, 816–827. [CrossRef]
39. Faul, F.; Erdfelder, E.; Lang, A.G.; Buchner, A. G*Power 3: A flexible statistical power analysis program for the social, behavioral, and biomedical sciences. *Behav. Res. Methods* **2007**, *39*, 175–191. [CrossRef]

40. Brucki, S.; Nitrini, R.; Caramelli, P.; Bertolucci, P.H.; Okamoto, I.H. Suggestions for utilization of the mini-mental state examination in Brazil. *Arq. Neuropsiquiatr.* **2003**, *61*, 777–781. [CrossRef]
41. Rose, D.J. *Fallproof!: A Comprehensive Balance and Mobility Training Program*, 2nd ed.; Human Kinetics: Champaign, IL, USA, 2010; ISBN 978-0-7360-6747-8.
42. Marfell-Jones, M.; Olds, T.; Stew, A.; Carter, L. *International Standards for Anthropometric Assessment*; International Society for the Advancement of Kinanthropometry: Wellington, New Zealand, 2018.
43. Creavin, S.T.; Noel-Storr, A.H.; Smailagic, N.; Giannakou, A.; Ewins, E.; Wisniewski, S.; Cullum, S. Mini-Mental State Examination (MMSE) for the detection of Alzheimer's dementia and other dementias in asymptomatic and previously clinically unevaluated people aged over 65 years in community and primary care populations. In *Cochrane Database of Systematic Reviews*; Creavin, S.T., Ed.; John Wiley & Sons, Ltd.: Chichester, UK, 2016.
44. Mazo, G.Z.; Mota, J.; Benedetti, T.B.; de Barros, M.V.G. Validade concorrente e reprodutibilidade: Teste-reteste do Questionário de Baecke modificado para idosos. *Rev. Bras. Atividade Física Saúde* **2001**, *6*, 5–11.
45. Voorrips, L.E.; Ravelli, A.C.; Dongelmans, P.C.; Deurenberg, P.A.U.L.; Van Staveren, W.A. A physical activity questionnaire for the elderly. *Med. Sci. Sport. Exerc.* **1991**, *23*, 974–979. [CrossRef]
46. Rikli, R.E.; Jones, C.J. Development and Validation of Criterion-Referenced Clinically Relevant Fitness Standards for Maintaining Physical Independence in Later Years. *Gerontologist* **2013**, *53*, 255–267. [CrossRef] [PubMed]
47. Cohen, J. Set correlation and contingency tables. *Appl. Psychol. Meas.* **1988**, *12*, 425–434. [CrossRef]
48. Preacher, K.J.; Rucker, D.D.; Hayes, A.F. Addressing Moderated Mediation Hypotheses: Theory, Methods, and Prescriptions. *Multivar. Behav. Res.* **2007**, *42*, 185–227. [CrossRef]
49. Hayes, A.F. *Introduction to Mediation, Moderation, and Conditional Process Analysis: A Regression-Based Approach*; Guilford Publications: New York, NY, USA, 2013; ISBN 978-1-60918-230-4.
50. WHO-World Health Organization Noncommunicable Diseases (NCD). Available online: https://www.who.int/gho/ncd/mortality_morbidity/en/ (accessed on 11 July 2022).
51. WHO-World Health Organization. *Noncommunicable Diseases Progress Monitor 2022*; WHO-World Health Organization: Geneva, Switzerland, 2022.
52. WHO-World Health Organization. *WHO Guidelines on Physical Activity and Sedentary Behaviour*; WHO-World Health Organization: Geneva, Switzerland, 2020; ISBN 9781134470006.
53. Liguori, G.; American College of Sports Medicine. *ACSM's Guidelines for Exercise Testing and Prescription*; Lippincott Williams & Wilkins: Philadelphia, PA, USA, 2020.
54. Hörder, H.; Skoog, I.; Frändin, K. Health-related quality of life in relation to walking habits and fitness: A population-based study of 75-year-olds. *Qual. Life Res.* **2013**, *22*, 1213–1223. [CrossRef] [PubMed]
55. Gomez-Bruton, A.; Navarrete-Villanueva, D.; Pérez-Gómez, J.; Vila-Maldonado, S.; Gesteiro, E.; Gusi, N.; Villa-Vicente, J.G.; Espino, L.; Gonzalez-Gross, M.; Casajus, J.A.; et al. The Effects of Age, Organized Physical Activity and Sedentarism on Fitness in Older Adults: An 8-Year Longitudinal Study. *Int. J. Environ. Res. Public Health* **2020**, *17*, 4312. [CrossRef]
56. Ferreira, M.L.; Sherrington, C.; Smith, K.; Carswell, P.; Bell, R.; Bell, M.; Nascimento, D.P.; Máximo Pereira, L.S.; Vardon, P. Physical activity improves strength, balance and endurance in adults aged 40–65 years: A systematic review. *J. Physiother.* **2012**, *58*, 145–156. [CrossRef]
57. Spartano, N.L.; Lyass, A.; Larson, M.G.; Tran, T.; Andersson, C.; Blease, S.J.; Esliger, D.W.; Vasan, R.S.; Murabito, J.M. Objective physical activity and physical performance in middle-aged and older adults. *Exp. Gerontol.* **2019**, *119*, 203–211. [CrossRef]
58. Amaral Gomes, E.S.; Ramsey, K.A.; Rojer, A.G.M.; Reijnierse, E.M.; Maier, A.B. The Association of Objectively Measured Physical Activity and Sedentary Behavior with (Instrumental) Activities of Daily Living in Community-Dwelling Older Adults: A Systematic Review. *Clin. Interv. Aging* **2021**, *16*, 1877–1915. [CrossRef]
59. Roberts, C.E.; Phillips, L.H.; Cooper, C.L.; Gray, S.; Allan, J.L. Effect of Different Types of Physical Activity on Activities of Daily Living in Older Adults: Systematic Review and Meta-Analysis. *J. Aging Phys. Act.* **2017**, *25*, 653–670. [CrossRef]
60. Perez-Sousa, M.A.; Venegas-Sanabria, L.C.; Chavarro-Carvajal, D.A.; Cano-Gutierrez, C.A.; Izquierdo, M.; Correa-Bautista, J.E.; Ramírez-Vélez, R. Gait speed used as a mediator of the effect of sarcopenia on dependency in activities of daily living. *J. Cachexia. Sarcopenia Muscle* **2019**, *10*, 1009–1015. [CrossRef]
61. Kiselev, J.; Nuritdinow, T.; Spira, D.; Buchmann, N.; Steinhagen-Thiessen, E.; Lederer, C.; Daumer, M.; Demuth, I. Long-term gait measurements in daily life: Results from the Berlin Aging Study II (BASE-II). *PLoS ONE* **2019**, *14*, e0225026. [CrossRef] [PubMed]
62. Shin, S.; Valentine, R.J.; Evans, E.M.; Sosnoff, J.J. Lower extremity muscle quality and gait variability in older adults. *Age Ageing* **2012**, *41*, 595–599. [CrossRef] [PubMed]
63. Ambrose, A.F.; Paul, G.; Hausdorff, J.M. Risk factors for falls among older adults: A review of the literature. *Maturitas* **2013**, *75*, 51–61. [CrossRef] [PubMed]
64. Allali, G.; Ayers, E.I.; Verghese, J. Multiple modes of assessment of gait are better than one to predict incident falls. *Arch. Gerontol. Geriatr.* **2015**, *60*, 389–393. [CrossRef]
65. Mielke, M.M.; Roberts, R.O.; Savica, R.; Cha, R.; Drubach, D.I.; Christianson, T.; Pankratz, V.S.; Geda, Y.E.; Machulda, M.M.; Ivnik, R.J.; et al. Assessing the Temporal Relationship Between Cognition and Gait: Slow Gait Predicts Cognitive Decline in the Mayo Clinic Study of Aging. *J. Gerontol. Ser. A Biol. Sci. Med. Sci.* **2013**, *68*, 929–937. [CrossRef] [PubMed]

66. Desai, P.; Evans, D.; Dhana, K.; Aggarwal, N.T.; Wilson, R.S.; McAninch, E.; Rajan, K.B. Longitudinal Association of Total Tau Concentrations and Physical Activity with Cognitive Decline in a Population Sample. *JAMA Netw. Open* **2021**, *4*, e2120398. [CrossRef]
67. Carvalho, A.; Rea, I.M.; Parimon, T.; Cusack, B.J. Physical activity and cognitive function in individuals over 60 years of age: A systematic review. *Clin. Interv. Aging* **2014**, *9*, 661–682.
68. Studenski, S.; Faulkner, K.; Inzitari, M.; Brach, J.; Chandler, J.; Cawthon, P.; Connor, E.B.; Kritchevsky, S.; Badinelli, S.; Harris, T.; et al. Gait Speed and Survival in Older Adults. *JAMA J. Am. Med. Assoc.* **2015**, *305*, 50–58. [CrossRef]
69. Rasmussen, L.J.H.; Caspi, A.; Ambler, A.; Broadbent, J.M.; Cohen, H.J.; D'Arbeloff, T.; Elliott, M.; Hancox, R.J.; Harrington, H.; Hogan, S.; et al. Association of Neurocognitive and Physical Function with Gait Speed in Midlife. *JAMA Netw. Open* **2019**, *2*, e1913123. [CrossRef]
70. White, D.K.; Neogi, T.; Nevitt, M.C.; Peloquin, C.E.; Zhu, Y.; Boudreau, R.M.; Cauley, J.A.; Ferrucci, L.; Harris, T.B.; Satterfield, S.M.; et al. Trajectories of Gait Speed Predict Mortality in Well-Functioning Older Adults: The Health, Aging and Body Composition Study. *J. Gerontol. Ser. A Biol. Sci. Med. Sci.* **2013**, *68*, 456–464. [CrossRef]
71. Galvão, L.L.; Silva, R.R.; Tribess, S.; Santos, D.A.T.; Junior, J.S.V. Physical activity combined with sedentary behaviour in the risk of mortality in older adults. *Rev. Saude Publica* **2021**, *55*, 60. [PubMed]
72. da Silva Sousa, N.F.; de Paule Barbosa Medina, L.; Bastos, T.F.; Monteiro, C.N.; Lima, M.G.; de Azevedo Barros, M.B. Social inequalities in the prevalence of indicators of active aging in the Brazilian population: National Health Survey, 2013. *Rev. Bras. Epidemiol.* **2019**, *22*.
73. Ribeiro, A.Q.; Salgado, S.M.L.; Gomes, I.S.; Fogal, A.S.; Martinho, K.O.; Almeida, L.F.F.; de Oliveira, W.C. Prevalence and factors associated with physical inactivity among the elderly: A population-based study. *Rev. Bras. Geriatr. Gerontol.* **2016**, *19*, 483–493. [CrossRef]
74. Dugan, S.A.; Gabriel, K.P.; Lange-Maia, B.S.; Karvonen-Gutierrez, C. Physical Activity and Physical Function. *Obstet. Gynecol. Clin. N. Am.* **2018**, *45*, 723–736. [CrossRef]
75. Manini, T.M.; Pahor, M. Physical activity and maintaining physical function in older adults. *Br. J. Sports Med.* **2008**, *43*, 28–31. [CrossRef] [PubMed]

Article

Interventions to Improve Physical Capability of Older Adults with Mild Disabilities: A Case Study

Cheng-En Wu [1], Kai Way Li [2,*], Fan Chia [3] and Wei-Yang Huang [4]

1. Ph.D. Program of Technology Management, Chung Hua University, Hsinchu 30012, Taiwan; d10903006@chu.edu.tw
2. Department of Industrial Management, Chung Hua University, Hsinchu 30012, Taiwan
3. Office of Physical Education and Sport, National Chung Hsin University, Taichung 40227, Taiwan; fan6423@nchu.edu.tw
4. National Taiwan College of Performing Arts, Taipei 11464, Taiwan; pmp999@tcpa.edu.tw
* Correspondence: kai@chu.edu.tw

Abstract: Ageing is related to changes in physical health, including loss of mobility and muscle function. It can lead to impaired physical capability and reduced quality of life. The purpose of this study was to investigate whether a physical activity rehabilitation program (PARP) could improve range of joint motion (ROM), grip strength, and gait speed of older adults with mild disabilities. Forty older adults in a long-term care center in Taiwan joined as human participants and were split into control and experimental groups. The participants in the experimental group joined a PARP for eight weeks. The ROM of bodily joints, grip strength, and gait speed of all participants were measured both before and after the eight-week period. The results showed that all the ROMs, grip strength, and gait speed of the participants in the experimental group increased significantly after attending the program. The improvement of the ROMs for male and female participants in the experimental group ranged from 3.8% to 71% and from 7.8% to 75%, respectively. Male participants had greater improvement on gait speed (50%) than their female counterparts (22.9%). Female participants, on the other hand, had greater improvement on grip strength (25.4%) than their male counterparts (20.3%). The ROM, grip strength, and gait speed of the control group, on the other hand, did not change significantly during the same period. The results showed that the PARP adopted in this study was effective in increasing the ROM, grip strength, and gait speed of those who had joined the PARP. This study shows that an eight-week PARP without the use of gym machines was beneficial in reducing sarcopenia in elderly people with mild disabilities.

Keywords: long-term care center; mildly disabled; rehabilitation; range of joint motion

1. Introduction

Ageing is a common phenomenon for both developed and developing countries. Due to the remarkable gain of life expectancy, older adult populations are growing rapidly [1]. Many older adults are losing their mental and/or physical functions and are becoming partially or totally disabled [2–4]. The need for long-term care for those individuals is becoming urgent. The literature has shown that in 2020 there were approximately half a million adults aged 65 or older with mild disabilities who needed long-term care in Taiwan [5]. The impaired body parts of those individuals may have limited mobility, weakness of muscular strength, and incapability to walk independently [6,7]. Performing activities of daily living (ADL) then becomes a problem for those adults [8,9].

Both the scales of ADL and instrumental activities of daily living (IADL) may be used to assess the level of bodily disabilities [10–12]. The ADL scale is used to measure the ability of a person performing the activities of daily living, such as bathing, dressing, eating, etc. An ADL score between 91 to 99 indicates a level of mildly disabled [10–12]. The IADL scale, on the other hand, assesses whether an individual may live independently with instrumental skills, such as being able to go shopping, do laundry, prepare food, complete household maintenance, and join outdoor activities. Those who need assistance with three out of the five items mentioned are considered mildly disabled [13].

Sarcopenia is common for older adults with mild disabilities. It may lead to slow walking, wheelchair walking, weakness, and tremors in upper limbs [14,15]. Sarcopenia is a muscle disease which is characterized by a loss of skeletal muscle mass and strength. It may lead to adverse outcomes such as physical disabilities, loss of capability in ADL, and even death [16–20]. Sarcopenia usually presents in a chronic and latent manner and increases gradually with age. It may also occur rapidly and is usually associated with acute immobility or serious illnesses such as prolonged hospitalization and disabilities [17,21–24]. The literature has proposed to diagnose upper limb sarcopenia via measuring the grip strength [23]. Male and female participants are diagnosed as having upper limb sarcopenia if their maximum grip strengths are lower than 26 and 18 kg, respectively. The gait speed, on the other hand, has been adopted to assess sarcopenia on lower limbs [25,26]. The literature [25] has ranked a walking speed less than 0.4 m/s, 0.4 to 0.8 m/s, 0.8 to 1.2 m/s, and 1.2 m/s or more as level 1, 2, 3, and 4, respectively, of sarcopenia. These four levels correspond to household ambulatory, limited community ambulatory, community ambulatory, and capability of crossing the street crossing, respectively.

People with mild disabilities may have impaired ADL capability and range of motion (ROM) of joints [25–30]. The ROM is the maximum arc of joint motion that can be achieved by a certain body part. Most people lose a certain amount of joint mobility as they age. This can be caused by muscle tightness, injury, pain, arthritis, or lack of exercise [31]. Disabled people suffer from degeneration or damage to ROM in some or all parts of the body, resulting in pain and stiffness that makes it difficult to squat, stand, walk, shower, dress, raise hands, and turn around. These limitations in motor control are attributed to deterioration in joint ROM. The extent to which a person with a disability can move a joint varies depending on the disabilities of the joint [32,33]. The gradual shrinkage of ROM is a signal that the body is deteriorating. Although ROM shrinkage does not constitute an injury, the loss of muscle mass over time due to limited mobility can lead to sarcopenia [15,17,34,35].

A physical activity rehabilitation program (PARP) is a program to assist people, especially those with a bodily disability, in improving the physical function of their bodies [26]. Such a program may include exercise training [27,28], muscular strength training [26], gait and balancing [24], and so on. It may increase the mobility of bodily joints and muscle strength and is important in helping people to restore their bodily function so as to live a better life. The literature [36] has indicated that the intensity of the training should be vigorous for a duration at least two months at a frequency of three training sessions per week [26,37]. Krist et al. [38], for example, conducted an eight-week rehabilitation program consisting of resistance training on 10 older participants (mean age 84 years) in a nursing home. Their training was performed using gym machines including chess press, rowing machine, butterfly reverse for the upper limbs, leg press and extension, and a crunch trainer for the abdominals. The training was twice per week and each session lasted for 45 min. They indicated that the training was effective in increasing the mobility and muscle strength of upper and lower limbs of their participants.

If elderly people are becoming disabled, their physical mobility will decline gradually, and they will be more likely to suffer sarcopenia. A PARP may improve the mobility of bodily joints and muscle strength to increase the physical capability of the partially disabled. There are examples showing that implementing a PARP improves the mobility and muscle strength of the participants [26,36,37]. However, the designs of the rehabilitation program and the outcomes among those examples might be quite different. More studies are required to examine the effects of a PARP on mitigating the sarcopenia of different older populations. In addition, many rehabilitation programs reported in the literature [36–38] relied on the use of gym machines. However, most nursing homes and long-term care centers in Taiwan do not have gym machines. Studies showing the effectiveness of a PARP without using those machines are required. The aim of this study was to provide such an example. In this study, a PARP without using gym machines was designed (see Section 2.2). The objective of this study was to show that such a program can be effective in mitigating the sarcopenia of the older participants with mild disabilities.

2. Materials and Methods

2.1. Participants

Forty older adults (20 males and 20 females) with mild disabilities [2,10–13] in the Cih-Pao Long-Term Care Center in Chiayi, Taiwan, joined our study as human participants. These adults were residents in the center. Ten male and ten female participants were assigned to each of the experimental and control groups randomly. The mean ages of male and female participants were 83.1 ($\pm$5.9) and 84.3 ($\pm$6.1) years, respectively. These participants could stand briefly but needed to be accompanied by a caregiver or use an assistive crutch to walk. They could wear and take off their clothes slowly on their own but needed caregivers to assist them in taking a bath (washing their hair and back which they were less capable of doing on their own). They could eat with a spoon but could not use chopsticks. Their mild disabilities were assessed by a rehabilitation physician of the center using both the ADL and IADL scales [2,9,10]. The algorithms for diagnosing sarcopenia in older adults in the literature [23] were adopted.

2.2. Physical Activity Rehabilitation Program

A PARP was developed in this study (see Table 1). This program involved physical activities at a moderate intensity lasting for 8 weeks and was implemented in the long-term care center under the supervision of a rehabilitation physician. The eight-week period followed recommendations in the literature [39]. According to the Center of Disease Control and Prevention (CDC) of the USA, moderate intensity implied that the heart rates of the participants were between 64% and 76% of their maximum heart rate [40]. The maximum heart rate was estimated using the 220 minus age equation. There were three sessions per week during weekdays [37]. Each session lasted for approximately 70 min with a one-minute break between courses (see Table 1). Each session started with lower and upper limb stretching, followed by seated knee raise, seated arm curl, seated stepping in place, seated hands touching one foot, seated shoulder and arm stretching, and finally seated back and pectoralis major stretching. All of the participants were diagnosed as having physical mobility impairments to a certain degree. These impairments were characterized by slow movement and functional limitations of ROM, resulting in partial ADL disability [9,10]. It was for this reason that all the courses in the training in Table 1 were performed while the participants were seated. All the participants in the experimental group joined this program. The participants in the control group, on the other hand, did not join this program. They lived as usual during the eight-week test period.

Table 1. Details of the PARP in this study.

Course	Posture and Motions	Operation Method
Lower body strength training	Seated (single) knee lift 12 (reps) × 5 (5 sets)	Sit with the body on two-thirds of the chair and lift one foot to the abdomen
Upper body strength training	Seated arm curl 12 (reps) × 5 (sets)	Stretch both arms forward and hold a water bottle (0.6 kg) to curl the biceps
Aerobic endurance training	3 min seated marching in place 3 min × 5 (sets)	Sit with two-thirds of the body on the chair, swing hands up and down on both sides of the chair, and step with the feet in place.
Stretching of lower limb	Seated with the back of the chair to extend the leg and ankle Left foot, right foot in turn 10 s × 12 (sets)	Raise one leg parallel to the ground, knee straight, tip the ankle up as far as possible, hold for 10 s
Stretching of upper limb	Seated shoulder and arm extensions for 10 s × 12 (sets) Seated back and pectoralis major extensions for 10 s × 12 (sets)	1. Cross both arms up and extend the shoulder joint to the highest point. 2. Extend both arms forward and outward on both sides of the body.

2.3. Apparatus and Measurements

The ROM assessments followed those in the literature [28,39]. The ROMs of both upper and lower extremities on the dominant side were measured both before and after the PARP. For the elbow and knee, the ROM of flexion was measured. For the wrist, both the ROMs of flexion and extension were measured. For the ankle, both the ROMs of plantarflexion and dorsiflexion were measured. The ROMs of both the abduction/protraction and adduction/retraction were measured for the hip. For the shoulder, the ROMs of flexion, extension, abduction, horizontal flexion, and horizontal extension were measured. The ROM values were measured using a goniometer (GemRed Inc., Guilin, China) (see Figure 1). The reading of the ROM was shown in a digital displayer.

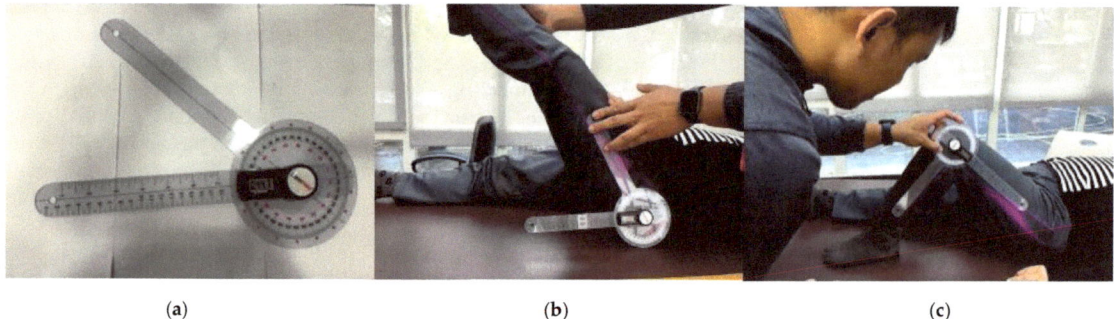

(a) (b) (c)

Figure 1. Goniometer and joint angle measurement: (a) goniometer; (b) hip range of motion measurement; (c) knee range of motion measurement.

The grip strengths of the dominant hand of the participants were measured both before and after the 8-week testing period to determine whether their grip strength had improved and thus their sarcopenia had ameliorated after they have joined the PARP. A dynamometer (EH101, Camry Electronic Co, Ltd., Zhongshan, China) (Table 2, Figure 2) was used for this purpose. This dynamometer could measure grip forces up to 90 kgf. The grip force reading was shown in a digital displayer. The grip span was 5 cm. When measuring this force, the participant stood erect with his or her arm straight down by the side. This posture was recommended by Li and Yu [41].

Table 2. Measurement of ROM, grip strength, and gait speed.

Assessment	Content
Range of Joint motion	1. Shoulder ROM: Flexion (0–180°), Extension (0–50°), Abduction (0–180°), Horizontal adduction (0–135°). 2. Elbow ROM: Flexion (0–150°). 3. Wrist ROM: Flexion (0–80°), Extension (0–80°). 4. Hip ROM: Flexion (0–100°), Extension (0–30°), Abduction/Protraction (0–40°), Abduction/Retraction (0–20°). 5. Knee ROM: Flexion (0–150°). 6. Ankle ROM: Plantarflexion (0–50°), Dorsiflexion (0–20°).
Sarcopenia	1. Measure the maximum grip strengths. 2. Measure the gait speed of a 12 m walk test on a flat walkway.

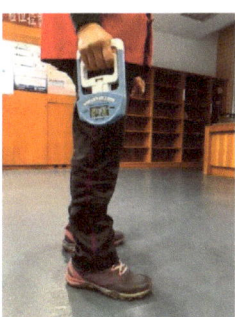

Figure 2. Grip strength measurement.

The gait speed of a 12-m walking test for all participants was measured to assess the sarcopenia of lower limbs both before and after the 8-week period [26]. A stopwatch was used to measure the time in this test.

2.4. Statistical Analysis

Descriptive statistics were performed. Shapiro–Wilk tests were performed for all the dependent variables for both male and female participants, for both control and experimental groups, and for both the pre-test and post-test data to check the normality assumption. The results showed that the hypothesis of normal distribution was supported for all the data. Pair-wised t-tests were performed to compare the pretest and posttest data of the participants and the difference between genders. Pearson's correlation coefficient between the ROM of the joints of upper limb and grip strength, and between the ROM of the joints of lower limb and gait speed of the experimental group, were calculated. The significance level of $\alpha = 0.05$ was adopted. The Cohen's d was calculated to determine the effect size of the t-tests and adequacy of sample size [42]. Statistical analyses were performed using the SPSS 20.0 software (IBM®, Armonk, NY, USA).

3. Results

All the participants in the experimental group completed the full eight-week program. There were no adverse effects of the program on the participants. The Cohen's d for all the dependent variables for the experimental group data ranged from 0.86 to 7.53, indicating large effect sizes [42]. Adopting a significance level of 0.05, a power of 0.8, and a sample size of 10 (for male and female participants in the experimental group), the Cohen's d should be 1.2 or higher. All the variables for each of the gender satisfied this level except the shoulder abduction for male participants (Cohen's d = 0.86). The adequacy of the sample size was therefore confirmed.

3.1. Range of Joint Motion

Tables 3 and 4 show the ROM results for male and female participants, respectively. After completing the PARP, the participants in the experimental group showed significant ($p < 0.05$) improvements in all the joint ROMs for both males and females. All the ROM values of the control group did not change significantly before and after the eight-week period. The most significant improvement for male participants in the experimental group joining the program was in the hip joint adduction/retraction which increased from 10.1° to 17.1°. This was an increase of 71%. The second most significant improvement (52.9%) of this group was the ROM of hip extension which increased from 18.3° to 26.1°. The improvement of the ROM of shoulder abduction of males, on the other hand, was the lowest (only 3.8%). For female participants, the leading improvement of the ROM was observed at the hip and the lowest improvement was the shoulder horizon extension and flexion (7.8%). These findings indicated that the participants experienced significant changes in the range of joint motion after joining the PARP. The eight-week PARP was effective in improving the ROMs for both male and female participants.

Table 3. ROM (°) of male participants before and after joining the PARP.

Body Part and Movement	Control Group (n = 10)			Experimental Group (n = 10)			Improvement (%)
	Pre-Test	Post-Test	p-Value	Pre-Test	Post-Test	p-Value	
Shoulder flexion	145.1 ± 12.6	145.2 ± 12.3	0.612	140.0 ± 12.5	157.0 ± 6.2	0.001	12.1
Shoulder extension	36.9 ± 4.9	37.0 ± 5.2	0.556	37.8 ± 3.9	42.8 ± 2.8	0.003	13.2
Shoulder abduction	136.4 ± 7.7	136.7 ± 7.4	0.134	140.8 ± 6.8	146.4 ± 6.2	0.002	3.8
Shoulder horizontal flexion/extension	113.2 ± 5.3	113.8 ± 5.4	0.068	115.4 ± 9.1	124.9 ± 7.2	0.001	8.7
Elbow flexion	122.4 ± 11.8	122.0 ± 11.6	0.093	122.4 ± 11.7	1439.7 ± 9.1	0.001	14.8
Wrist flexion	66.4 ± 3.8	66.2 ± 3.7	0.083	64.0 ± 4.3	70.2 ± 4.9	0.003	9.4
Wrist extension	60.3 ± 3.1	60.9 ± 2.7	0.058	60.2 ± 2.6	67.1 ± 2.3	0.002	11.7
Hip flexion	67.6 ± 9.7	67.2 ± 9.9	0.112	67.6 ± 9.8	75.6 ± 10.6	0.004	11.8
Hip extension	18.2 ± 3.2	18.1 ± 3.2	0.574	18.3 ± 3.1	26.1 ± 3.0	0.001	52.9
Hip abduction/protraction	31.1 ± 2.4	31.2 ± 2.6	0.327	33.5 ± 3.2	42.1 ± 1.5	0.003	27.3
Hip adduction/retraction	10.2 ± 1.5	10.3 ± 1.6	0.276	10.1 ± 2.1	17.1 ± 2.3	0.001	71
Knee flexion	93.2 ± 8.4	94.6 ± 8.2	0.557	97.1 ± 8.4	114.9 ± 8.2	0.001	23.5
Ankle plantarflexion	35.7 ± 3.5	36.4 ± 3.4	0.077	35.9 ± 3.7	42.6 ± 2.1	0.003	19.4
Ankle dorsiflexion	8.5 ± 1.8	8.4 ± 1.5	0.486	9.1 ± 1.9	12.6 ± 1.9	0.001	44.4

Values are presented as means ± standard deviations; improvement = (post − pre)/pre × 100% for the experimental group.

Table 4. ROM (°) of female participants before and after joining the PARP.

Body Part and Movement	Control Group (n = 10)			Experimental Group (n = 10)			Improvement (%)
	Pre-Test	Post-Test	p-Value	Pre-Test	Post-Test	p-Value	
Shoulder flexion	139.1 ± 11.4	139.0 ± 11.5	0.449	139.4 ± 9.8	158.8 ± 7.5	0.001	13.6
Shoulder extension	36.6 ± 5.2	36.3 ± 5.5	0.437	37.2 ± 6.2	42.7 ± 4.1	0.007	16.2
Shoulder abduction	137.7 ± 7.4	138.5 ± 7.7	0.086	137.9 ± 8.4	152.3 ± 3.4	0.004	10.4
Shoulder horizontal flexion/extension	118.6 ± 9.3	118.8 ± 9.2	0.257	115.8 ± 6.6	125.0 ± 5.0	0.008	7.8
Elbow flexion	108.9 ± 10.4	108.7 ± 10.0	0.362	110.2 ± 10.4	141.9 ± 5.0	0.003	29.1
Wrist flexion	58.8 ± 3.0	58.7 ± 3.1	0.163	57.8 ± 4.2	67.4 ± 4.0	0.004	15.5
Wrist extension	60.1 ± 2.6	60.4 ± 2.8	0.059	60.2 ± 2.4	67.9 ± 1.8	0.001	13.3
Hip flexion	60.8 ± 11.7	60.5 ± 11.6	0.485	60.4 ± 11.6	72.4 ± 8.1	0.002	20.0
Hip extension	18.9 ± 2.8	19.1 ± 2.47	0.313	18.4 ± 2.9	25.9 ± 2.1	0.001	44.4
Hip abduction/protraction	33.8 ± 3.7	33.9 ± 3.8	0.868	32.5 ± 2.6	40.5 ± 3.3	0.004	24.2
Hip adduction/retraction	10.3 ± 1.6	10.2 ± 1.4	0.513	10.2 ± 1.5	17.5 ± 2.1	0.001	75.0
Knee flexion	105.3 ± 4.1	105.7 ± 3.9	0.121	105.1 ± 3.3	120.8 ± 2.6	0.001	15.0
Ankle plantarflexion	36.1 ± 4.7	36.2 ± 4.7	0.717	35.6 ± 4.4	42.9 ± 2.5	0.001	22.9
Ankle dorsiflexion	9.2 ± 1.5	9.1 ± 1.2	0.375	8.9 ± 1.2	13.6 ± 1.8	0.003	75.0

Values are presented as means ± standard deviations; improvement = (post − pre)/pre × 100% for the experimental group.

Comparisons of the ROM values between male and female participants in the experimental group after attending the PARP (Tables 3 and 4) showed that females had significantly ($p < 0.05$) higher ROMs in both shoulder abduction (152.3 ± 3.4°) and hip adduction/retraction (17.5 ± 2.1°) than those of males (146.4 ± 6.2° and 17.1 ± 2.3°, respectively). The ROM of knee flexion for females in the experimental group after attending the PARP (120.8 ± 2.6°) was also significantly higher (114.9 ± 8.2°) than that of males ($p < 0.05$). No significant differences between males and females were found on other ROM values.

3.2. Grip Strength and Gait Speed

The grip strength and gait speed for both males and females in the experimental group after attending the PARP were significantly higher than those before the program (see

Table 5). The mean grip strength for male and female participants increased from 7.1 kgf to 8.6 kgf ($p < 0.05$) and from 6.0 kgf to 7.6 kgf ($p < 0.05$), respectively. The improvement of grip strength of female and male participants was 25.4% and 20.3%, respectively. The mean gait speed of male and female participants of the experimental group increased from 0.4 m/s to 0.6 m/s ($p < 0.05$) and from 0.5 m/s to 0.6 m/s ($p < 0.05$), respectively. Male participants in the experimental group had greater improvement (50.0%) on gait speed after attending the PARP than that of their male counterparts (22.9%). In addition, the gait speeds for both male and female participants in the control group before and after the eight-week period were not significantly different. This implied that older adults showed significant improvement in sarcopenia in terms of grip strength and walking speed after joining the PARP.

Table 5. Comparisons of grip strength and gait speed before and after the PARP.

Variables	Control Group ($n = 10$)			Experimental Group ($n = 10$)			Improvement (%)
	Pre-Test	Post-Test	p-Value	Pre-Test	Post-Test	p-Value	
Males HS (kgf)	6.2 ± 0.9	6.3 ± 0.9	0.085	7.1 ± 0.5	8.6 ± 0.6	0.001	20.3
Females HS (kgf)	6.0 ± 0.6	6.0 ± 0.7	0.432	6.0 ± 0.8	7.6 ± 1.1	0.003	25.4
Males GS (m/s)	0.4 ± 0.1	0.4 ± 0.1	0.057	0.4 ± 0.1	0.6 ± 0.1	0.004	50.0
Females GS (m/s)	0.5 ± 0.1	0.5 ± 0.1	0.109	0.5 ± 0.1	0.6 ± 0.1	0.004	22.9

HS: grip strength, GS: gait speed; values are mean ± standard deviation; improvement = (post − pre)/pre × 100% for the experimental group.

Table 6 shows the correlation coefficients between the ROM of the upper extremities and grip strength and between the ROM of the lower extremities and gait speed that were higher than 0.6 ($p < 0.0001$). These results showed that the changes of ROM were significantly associated with the mitigation of sarcopenia in terms of grip strength and gait speed after joining the PARP.

Table 6. Correlation analysis between the range of motion of upper and lower limbs and handgrip strength and gait speed.

Improvement (%)	SF	EF	WF	WE	HF	HE	KF	AP	AD
Males HS	0.77 *	0.87 *	0.72 *	0.65 *	-	-	-	-	-
Females HS	0.73 *	0.75 *	0.83 *	0.77 *	-	-	-	-	-
Males GS	-	-	-	-	0.62 *	0.69 *	0.81 *	0.66 *	0.69 *
Females GS	-	-	-	-	0.67 *	0.65 *	0.82 *	0.62 *	0.74 *

* $p < 0.05$; HS: grip strength; GS: gait speed; SF: shoulder flexion, EF: elbow flexion, WF: wrist flexion, WE: wrist extension, HF: hip flexion, HE: hip extension, KF: knee flexion, AP: ankle plantarflexion, AD: ankle dorsiflexion.

4. Discussion

People with mild disabilities generally have a gradual decline in joint mobility [43–45]. The mean age of our participants was approximately 84 years old. These participants nearly all belonged to the oldest group as categorized in the literature [46]. The literature has shown that ROM is negatively correlated with disabilities [47–51]. Improvements in ROM may then imply improvement of disability. All the ROMs of the participants in the experimental groups increased after they had completed the PARP (Tables 3 and 4). This implies that the program adopted in the current study was effective in increasing the mobility of the joints measured and hence was helpful in reducing mobility impairments. The physiotherapist and physical activity trainers in the current study assisted the older adults in performing stretching and plyometric exercises in a seated position. We found that after these exercises, not only did the ROM values increase, but also the speeds of movement of both upper and lower limbs. Upon completing the program, the participants could get up from a chair, step in place, and walk faster than they previously could [14]. These findings provide important information about ROM and muscle strength generation.

Shoulder and trunk inflexibility is common for older adults. Declines of elbow and knee dexterity are relatively less common. After attending the program adopted in this study, both male and female participants in the experimental groups made significant progress on both the adduction/retraction and extension of the hip. These improvements could be attributed to our training involving the lower limbs as there was no trunk muscle training in the program in Table 1. This was consistent with that of Roaas and Andersson [52]. It also implies that the lower limb training in the current study helped in increasing hip mobility.

Declines of both muscle strength and gait speed are indicators of sarcopenia [23]. The literature suggests that grip strength is an indicator of overall muscle strength [41]. Both grip strength and gait speed have been recommended to assess the onset of sarcopenia. The grip strength of male and female participants in the experimental group increased 20.3% and 25.4%, respectively, after completing the program. This implies that the strength training on the upper body adopted in this study was effective in increasing the grip strength for the participants. This increase might be attributed to the increase of muscle mass on their upper limbs. Such an increase was evidence of the mitigation of sarcopenia on the upper limbs for the participants. Increase of grip strength is important for older adults, especially for those with mild disabilities. It may increase their capabilities in ADL, such as eating and dressing on their own.

The gait speeds of the participants in the control group had negligible changes during the eight-week period of the study. They were significantly ($p < 0.05$) slower than those of the experimental group after attending the program in Table 1. The gait speed of the male and female participants who had joined the PARP increased 50% and 22.9%, respectively, after completing the program. Three of the male participants in the experimental group were in level 1 (household ambulatory) sarcopenia [43,53] before joining the rehabilitation program. They were advanced to level 2 (limited community ambulatory) after completing the program. This implies that the training adopted in this study on lower limbs was effective in promoting lower limb mobility. This improvement was evident in terms of the ROMs of the lower limbs and their gait speed. This also indicates the mitigation of sarcopenia on lower limbs among those participants [44]. Male participants gained more gait speed than their female counterparts after attending the program, indicating our training on lower limbs was more effective on males than on females.

Older adults with mild disabilities have inherent impairments in voluntary mobility and age-related declines in musculoskeletal function, resulting in frailty and loss of independence. This study indicates that the PARP in Table 1 was effective in increasing joint ROM and mitigating the decline of sarcopenia. Sustained physical activity rehabilitation could also improve the gait speed of older adults with mild disabilities and reintegrate them into community life. The PARP adopted in this study does not require gym machines. It may be reproduced in other long-term care centers to improve the physical capability of older adults with mild disabilities.

The PARP adopted in the literature [38,54] utilized gym machines to assist the older adults in strengthening their physical capability during a period of 4 to 12 weeks. In the current study, simple exercises without using gym machines were performed for a period of eight weeks. The similarities of the former literature and our study were that the age groups of the participants were similar and both the former and later all led to the conclusion that the PARP was beneficial on the mobility and physical capability of the older adults. However, there were discrepancies between the current study and the literature mentioned. The results in the current study where females gained significantly more improvement on three of their ROMs than males were inconsistent with that in Krist et al. [38] where they found the improvement of mobility of males was greater than females. The grip strength improvement of male and female participants upon attending the PARP in the current study was 20.3% and 25.4%, respectively. These were higher than (11%) in Cadore et al. [26] and were lower than (33%) in Meuleman et al. [54]. These discrepancies might be attributed to the difference among the PARP adopted in different studies. They might also be attributed to the difference in racial groups (participants from Spain [26], Germany [38], and USA [54] versus Taiwan) among these studies.

There are limitations of this study. The first one was that all the participants were residences of the same long-term care center. The sample in this study was a convenient sample. The sample size was subjected to the limitation of the long-term care center population. The sample might not be representative of the general population of older adults. The second was that the participants in the control groups received no extra activity even if they were included in this study. The training intervention could have provided stimulation that resulted in a nonspecific benefit to the participants in the experimental group because of their awareness of the existence of the control group. This could have a confounding effect on the results of the PARP adopted in this study. This should be considered when interpreting the results of this study.

5. Conclusions

Muscle strength, gait speed, and ROM of the joints are important indicators of daily living function for older adults. These physical parameters may be improved via a properly designed physical rehabilitation program. In this study, a PARP without using any gym machines and lasting for eight weeks was designed and implemented for the older adults with mild disabilities in a long-term care center. The results showed that the program was effective in increasing the ROM of all joints tested, grip strength, and gait speed for those who joined the program. The difference of the ROM improvements between male and female participants was, however, insignificant. The benefits of joining such a program included increased mobility and mitigation of sarcopenia for the participants.

Author Contributions: Conceptualization, K.W.L. and C.-E.W.; methodology, W.-Y.H. and F.C.; software, C.-E.W.; validation, F.C. and C.-E.W.; formal analysis, K.W.L.; investigation, F.C.; resources, K.W.L.; data curation, W.-Y.H. and C.-E.W.; writing—original draft preparation, W.-Y.H.; writing—review and editing, K.W.L., C.-E.W. and W.-Y.H.; supervision, K.W.L. All authors have read and agreed to the published version of the manuscript.

Funding: This research received no external funding.

Institutional Review Board Statement: The study was conducted according to the guidelines of the Declaration of Helsinki and was approved by a local Institutional Review Board (Jen-Ai hospital 110-86).

Informed Consent Statement: Informed consent was obtained from all the participants in the study.

Data Availability Statement: Data available upon request.

Acknowledgments: This study was supported by the Cibao long-term care center in Chiayi County, Taiwan. The authors thank the rehabilitation physicians, nurses, and physical activity trainers at the center for their assistance in this study. The authors also thank the participants who voluntarily joined the study.

Conflicts of Interest: The authors declare no conflict of interest.

References

1. OECD/WHO. Ratio of people aged 15-64 to people aged over 65 years, 2020 and 2050. In *Health at a Glance: Asia/Pacific 2020: Measuring Progress towards Universal Health Coverage*; OECD Publishing: Paris, France, 2020. [CrossRef]
2. Ćwirlej-Sozańska, A.; Wiśniowska-Szurlej, A.; Wilmowska-Pietruszyńska, A.; Sozański, B. Determinants of ADL and IADL disability in older adults in southeastern Poland. *BMC Geriatr.* **2019**, *19*, 297. [CrossRef] [PubMed]
3. Zhang, W.; Feldman, M.W. Disability trajectories in activities of daily living of elderly Chinese before death. *China Popul. Dev. Stud.* **2020**, *4*, 127–151. [CrossRef]
4. Filippi, M.; Bar-Or, A.; Piehl, F.; Preziosa, P.; Solari, A.; Vukusic, S.; Rocca, M.A. Multiple sclerosis. *Nat. Rev. Dis. Primers* **2018**, *4*, 43. [CrossRef] [PubMed]
5. Wu, K.F.; Hu, J.L.; Chiou, H. Degrees of shortage and uncovered ratios for long-term care in Taiwan's regions: Evidence from dynamic DEA. *Int. J. Environ. Res. Public Health* **2021**, *18*, 605. [CrossRef]
6. Hsu, E.; Cohen, S.P. Postamputation pain: Epidemiology, mechanisms, and treatment. *J. Pain Res.* **2013**, *6*, 121–136. [CrossRef]

7. Hirani, V.; Blyth, F.; Naganathan, V.; Le Couteur, D.G.; Seibel, M.J.; Waite, L.M.; Handelsman, D.J.; Cumming, R.G. Sarcopenia is associated with incident disability, institutionalization, and mortality in community-dwelling older men: The concord health and ageing in men project. *J. Am. Med. Dir. Assoc.* **2015**, *16*, 607–613. [CrossRef] [PubMed]
8. Adekoya, A.A.; Guse, L. Wandering behavior from the perspectives of older adults with mild to moderate dementia in long-term care. *Res. Gerontol. Nurs.* **2019**, *12*, 239–247. [CrossRef]
9. Tabira, T.; Hotta, M.; Murata, M.; Yoshiura, K.; Han, G.; Ishikawa, T.; Koyama, A.; Ogawa, N.; Maruta, M.; Ikeda, Y.; et al. Age-related changes in instrumental and basic activities of daily living impairment in older adults with very mild Alzheimer's disease. *Dement. Geriatr. Cogn. Disord. Extra* **2020**, *10*, 27–37. [CrossRef] [PubMed]
10. Phelan, E.A.; Williams, B.; Penninx, B.W.; LoGerfo, J.P.; Leveille, S.G. Activities of daily living function and disability in older adults in a randomized trial of the health enhancement program. *J. Gerontol. A Biol. Sci. Med. Sci.* **2004**, *59*, 838–843. [CrossRef]
11. He, S.; Craig, B.A.; Xu, H.; Covinsky, K.E.; Stallard, E.; Thomas, J., 3rd; Hass, Z.; Sands, L.P. Unmet need for ADL assistance is associated with mortality among older adults with mild disability. *J. Gerontol. A Biol. Sci. Med. Sci.* **2015**, *70*, 1128–1132. [CrossRef] [PubMed]
12. Iwaya, T.; Doi, T.; Seichi, A.; Hoshino, Y.; Ogata, T.; Akai, M. Characteristics of disability in activity of daily living in elderly people associated with locomotive disorders. *BMC Geriatr.* **2017**, *17*, 165. [CrossRef]
13. Liao, W.L.; Chang, Y.H. Age trajectories of disability in instrumental activities of daily living and disability-free life expectancy among middle-aged and older adults in Taiwan: An 11-year longitudinal study. *BMC Geriatr.* **2020**, *20*, 530. [CrossRef]
14. Kim, M.; Won, C.W. Sarcopenia is associated with cognitive impairment mainly due to slow gait speed: Results from the Korean frailty and aging cohort study (KFACS). *Int. J. Environ. Res. Public Health* **2019**, *16*, 1491. [CrossRef]
15. Mile, M.; Balogh, L.; Papp, G.; Pucsok, J.M.; Szabó, L.; Barna, L.; Csiki, Z.; Lekli, I. Effects of functional training on sarcopenia in elderly women in the presence or absence of ACE inhibitors. *Int. J. Environ. Res. Public Health* **2021**, *18*, 6594. [CrossRef] [PubMed]
16. Beaudart, C.; Rizzoli, R.; Bruyère, O.; Reginster, J.Y.; Biver, E. Sarcopenia: Burden and challenges for public health. *Arch. Public Health* **2014**, *72*, 45. [CrossRef]
17. Bravo-José, P.; Moreno, E.; Espert, M.; Romeu, M.; Martínez, P.; Navarro, C. Prevalence of sarcopenia and associated factors in institutionalised older adult patients. *Clin. Nutr. ESPEN* **2018**, *27*, 113–119. [CrossRef] [PubMed]
18. Cruz-Jentoft, A.J.; Bahat, G.; Bauer, J.; Boirie, Y.; Bruyère, O.; Cederholm, T.; Cooper, C.; Landi, F.; Rolland, Y.; Sayer, A.A.; et al. Sarcopenia: Revised European consensus on definition and diagnosis. *Age Ageing* **2019**, *48*, 16–31. [CrossRef]
19. Chen, L.K.; Liu, L.K.; Woo, J.; Assantachai, P.; Auyeung, T.W.; Bahyah, K.S.; Chou, M.Y.; Chen, L.Y.; Hsu, P.S.; Krairit, O.; et al. Sarcopenia in Asia: Consensus report of the Asian Working Group for sarcopenia. *J. Am. Med. Dir. Assoc.* **2014**, *15*, 95–101. [CrossRef]
20. Studenski, S.A.; Peters, K.W.; Alley, D.E.; Cawthon, P.M.; McLean, R.R.; Harris, T.B.; Ferrucci, L.; Guralnik, J.M.; Fragala, M.S.; Kenny, A.M.; et al. The FNIH sarcopenia project: Rationale, study description, conference recommendations, and final estimates. *J. Gerontol. A Biol. Sci. Med. Sci.* **2014**, *69*, 547–558. [CrossRef]
21. Welch, C.; Hassan-Smith, Z.K.; Greig, C.A.; Lord, J.M.; Jackson, T.A. Acute sarcopenia secondary to hospitalization—An emerging condition affecting older adults. *Aging Dis.* **2018**, *9*, 151–164. [CrossRef] [PubMed]
22. Morley, J.E.; von Haehling, S.; Anker, S.D.; Vellas, B. From sarcopenia to frailty: A road less traveled. *J. Cachexia Sarcopenia Muscle* **2014**, *5*, 5–8. [CrossRef] [PubMed]
23. Rodriguez-Rejon, A.I.; Artacho, R.; Puerta, A.; Zuñiga, A.; Ruiz-Lopez, M.D. Diagnosis of sarcopenia in long-term care homes for the elderly: The sensitivity and specificity of two simplified algorithms with respect to the EWGSOP consensus. *J. Nutr. Health Aging* **2018**, *22*, 796–801. [CrossRef]
24. Roquebert, Q.; Sicsic, J.; Santos-Eggimann, B.; Sirven, N.; Rapp, T. Frailty, sarcopenia and long term care utilization in older populations: A systematic review. *J. Frailty Aging* **2021**, *10*, 272–280. [CrossRef] [PubMed]
25. Peel, N.M.; Kuys, S.S.; Klein, K. Gait speed as a measure in geriatric assessment in clinical settings: A systematic review. *J. Gerontol. A Biol. Sci. Med. Sci.* **2013**, *68*, 39–46. [CrossRef]
26. Cadore, E.L.; Casas-Herrero, A.; Zambom-Ferraresi, F.; Idoate, F.; Millor, N.; Gómez, M.; Rodríguez-Mañas, L.; Izquierdo, M. Multicomponent exercises including muscle power training enhance muscle mass, power output, and functional outcomes in institutionalized frail nonagenarians. *Age* **2014**, *36*, 773–785. [CrossRef] [PubMed]
27. Cooney, J.K.; Law, R.J.; Matschke, V.; Lemmey, A.B.; Moore, J.P.; Ahmad, Y.; Jones, J.G.; Maddison, P.; Thom, J.M. Benefits of exercise in rheumatoid arthritis. *J. Aging Res.* **2011**, *2011*, 681640. [CrossRef]
28. de Souto Barreto, P.; Morley, J.E.; Chodzko-Zajko, W.H.; Pitkala, K.; Weening-Djiksterhuis, E.; Rodriguez-Mañas, L.; Barbagallo, M.; Rosendahl, E.; Sinclair, A.; Landi, F.; et al. Recommendations on physical activity and exercise for older adults living in long-term care facilities: A taskforce report. *J. Am. Med. Dir. Assoc.* **2016**, *17*, 381–392. [CrossRef]
29. Svensson, M.; Lind, V.; Löfgren Harringe, M. Measurement of knee joint range of motion with a digital goniometer: A reliability study. *Physiother. Res. Int.* **2019**, *24*, e1765. [CrossRef]
30. Buchman, A.S.; Leurgans, S.E.; Wang, T.; Schnaider-Beeri, M.; Agarwal, P.; Dawe, R.J.; Delbono, O.; Bennett, D.A. Motor function is the primary driver of the associations of sarcopenia and physical frailty with adverse health outcomes in community-dwelling older adults. *PLoS ONE* **2021**, *16*, e0245680. [CrossRef] [PubMed]
31. Ferreira, F.G.; Juvanhol, L.L.; Silva-Costa, A.; Longo, G.Z. The mediating role of visceral adiposity in the relationship among schooling, physical inactivity, and unhealthy metabolic phenotype. *Am. J. Hum. Biol.* **2020**, *32*, e23425. [CrossRef] [PubMed]

32. Valamatos, M.J.; Tavares, F.; Santos, R.M.; Veloso, A.P.; Mil-Homens, P. Influence of full range of motion vs. equalized partial range of motion training on muscle architecture and mechanical properties. *Eur. J. Appl. Physiol.* **2018**, *118*, 1969–1983. [CrossRef] [PubMed]
33. Valderrabano, V.; Steiger, C. Treatment and prevention of osteoarthritis through exercise and sports. *J. Aging Res.* **2011**, *2011*, 374653. [CrossRef]
34. Angulo, J.; El Assar, M.; Álvarez-Bustos, A.; Rodríguez-Mañas, L. Physical activity and exercise: Strategies to manage frailty. *Redox. Biol.* **2020**, *35*, 101513. [CrossRef] [PubMed]
35. Janssen, I. Influence of sarcopenia on the development of physical disability: The cardiovascular health study. *J. Am. Geriatr. Soc.* **2006**, *54*, 56–62. [CrossRef]
36. Valenzuela, T. Efficacy of progressive resistance training interventions in older adults in nursing homes: A systematic review. *J. Am. Med. Dir. Assoc.* **2012**, *13*, 418–428. [CrossRef] [PubMed]
37. Venturelli, M.; Lanza, M. Positive effects of physical training in activity of daily living-dependent older adults. *Exp. Aging Res.* **2010**, *36*, 190–205. [CrossRef]
38. Krist, L.; Dimeo, F.; Keil, T. Can progressive resistance training twice a week improve mobility, muscle strength, and quality of life in very elderly nursing-home residents with impaired mobility? A pilot study. *Clin. Interv. Aging* **2013**, *8*, 443. [CrossRef]
39. Larsson, L.; Degens, H.; Li, M.; Salviati, L.; Lee, Y.I.; Thompson, W.; Kirkland, J.L.; Sandri, M. Sarcopenia: Aging-related loss of muscle mass and function. *Physiol. Rev.* **2019**, *99*, 427–511. [CrossRef]
40. Centers for Disease Control and Prevention, USA, Target Heart Rate and Estimated Maximum Heart Rate. Available online: https://www.cdc.gov/physicalactivity/basics/measuring/heartrate.htm (accessed on 18 January 2022).
41. Li, K.W.; Yu, R.-f. Assessment of grip force and subjective hand force exertion under handedness and postural conditions. *Appl. Ergon.* **2011**, *42*, 929–933. [CrossRef] [PubMed]
42. Cohen, J. *Statistical Power Analysis for the Behavioural Sciences*, 2nd ed.; Hillside: New York, NY, USA, 1988; pp. 20–26.
43. Soucie, J.M.; Wang, C.; Forsyth, A.; Funk, S.; Denny, M.; Roach, K.E.; Boone, D.; Hemophilia Treatment Center Network. Range of motion measurements: Reference values and a database for comparison studies. *Haemophilia* **2011**, *17*, 500–507. [CrossRef] [PubMed]
44. Dodge, H.H.; Kadowaki, T.; Hayakawa, T.; Yamakawa, M.; Sekikawa, A.; Ueshima, H. Cognitive impairment as a strong predictor of incident disability in specific ADL-IADL tasks among community-dwelling elders: The Azuchi study. *Gerontologist* **2005**, *45*, 222–230. [CrossRef] [PubMed]
45. Medeiros, H.B.; de Araújo, D.S.; de Araújo, C.G. Age-related mobility loss is joint-specific: An analysis from 6000 Flexitest results. *Age* **2013**, *35*, 2399–2407. [CrossRef] [PubMed]
46. Christensen, K.; Doblhammer, G.; Rau, R.; Vaupel, J.W. Ageing populations: The challenges ahead. *Lancet* **2009**, *74*, 1196–1208. [CrossRef]
47. Jung, H.; Yamasaki, M. Association of lower extremity range of motion and muscle strength with physical performance of community-dwelling older women. *J. Physiol. Anthropol.* **2016**, *35*, 30. [CrossRef] [PubMed]
48. Steultjens, M.P.; Dekker, J.; van Baar, M.E.; Oostendorp, R.A.; Bijlsma, J.W. Range of joint motion and disability in patients with osteoarthritis of the knee or hip. *Rheumatology* **2000**, *39*, 955–961. [CrossRef] [PubMed]
49. Beissner, K.L.; Collins, J.E.; Holmes, H. Muscle force and range of motion as predictors of function in older adults. *Phys. Ther.* **2000**, *80*, 556–563. [CrossRef]
50. Bello, A.I.; Ababio, E.; Antwi-Baffoe, S.; Seidu, M.A.; Adjei, D.N. Pain, range of motion and activity level as correlates of dynamic balance among elderly people with musculoskeletal disorder. *Ghana Med. J.* **2014**, *48*, 214–218. [CrossRef] [PubMed]
51. Menz, H.B. Biomechanics of the ageing foot and ankle: A mini-review. *Gerontology* **2015**, *61*, 381–388. [CrossRef]
52. Roaas, A.; Andersson, G.B. Normal range of motion of the hip, knee and ankle joints in male subjects, 30-40 years of age. *Acta Orthop. Scand.* **1982**, *53*, 205–208. [CrossRef] [PubMed]
53. Hai, S.; Wang, H.; Cao, L.; Liu, P.; Zhou, J.; Yang, Y.; Dong, B. Association between sarcopenia with lifestyle and family function among community-dwelling Chinese aged 60 years and older. *BMC Geriatr.* **2017**, *17*, 187. [CrossRef] [PubMed]
54. Meuleman, J.R.; Brechue, W.F.; Kubilis, P.S.; Lowenthal, D.T. Exercise Training in the debilitated aged: Strength and functional outcomes. *Arch. Phys. Med. Rehabil.* **2000**, *81*, 312–318. [CrossRef]

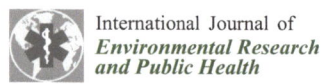 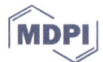

Article

Functional Capacity of Tai Chi-Practicing Elderly People

Alba Niño *, José Gerardo Villa-Vicente and Pilar S. Collado

Institute of Biomedicine (IBIOMED), University of Leon, 24071 Leon, Spain; jg.villa@unileon.es (J.G.V.-V.); mpsanc@unileon.es (P.S.C.)
* Correspondence: albaninogonzalez@gmail.com; Tel.: +34-626-014-644

Abstract: Research shows that ageing is modifiable or modulable, attending to external modifications and lifestyle factors: physical activity has a unique contribution to functional health and energy balance. Extensive research shows Tai Chi (TC) produced a major physical condition. To determine the impact of lifestyle on functional capacity, comparing the impact of continued long-life practice. 113 individuals (±71.53 years old): (a) PTC (n = 27); senior competitors, life-long training; (b) TC (n = 27); ±4 years; (c) Keep-Fit (KF n = 36); ±4 years; and the control group (d) sedentary individuals (SI n = 23). Five tests from the Senior Fitness Test (SFT) were used to assess the physical condition. The TC group showed significantly better results than the KF group: 30-s chair stand (23.22 ± 3.08 * rep vs. 17.17 ± 2.96 rep), chair sit-and-reach (2.19 ± 4.85 * cm vs. −1.93 ± 5.46 cm) and back scratch (1.02 ± 4.46 * cm vs. −2.43 ± 5.78 cm). The TCP group showed better results than the TC group: 30-s chair stand (27.70 ± 4.98 * rep vs. 23.22 ± 3.08 rep), 30-s arm curl (30.22 ± 4.36 * rep vs. 23.48 ± 3.42 rep), chair sit-and-reach (13.07 ± 4.00 * cm vs. 2.19 ± 4.85 cm) and back scratch (5.48 ± 3.51 * cm vs. 1.02 ± 4.46 cm). Among the different activities analysed, TC showed better results in SFT tests; in particular considering the long-life training of this martial art.

Keywords: aging; physical activity; Tai Chi; Chinese; physical fitness

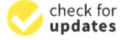

Citation: Niño, A.; Villa-Vicente, J.G.; S. Collado, P. Functional Capacity of Tai Chi-Practicing Elderly People. *Int. J. Environ. Res. Public Health* **2022**, *19*, 2178. https://doi.org/10.3390/ijerph19042178

Academic Editors: Andy Pringle and Nicola Kime

Received: 11 January 2022
Accepted: 11 February 2022
Published: 15 February 2022

Publisher's Note: MDPI stays neutral with regard to jurisdictional claims in published maps and institutional affiliations.

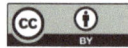

Copyright: © 2022 by the authors. Licensee MDPI, Basel, Switzerland. This article is an open access article distributed under the terms and conditions of the Creative Commons Attribution (CC BY) license (https://creativecommons.org/licenses/by/4.0/).

1. Introduction

Ageing is a life-long process that may imply a progressive loss of physical fitness. Older persons are typically physically inactive and spend more time in sedentary behaviours; it is necessary to emphasise the importance of physical fitness, health and independence for as many years as possible, adapted explicitly to this group [1].

A sedentary lifestyle has detrimental effects and physical consequences for older adults' health. Inactivity accentuates the progressive loss of autonomy and quality of life of older people at an alarming rate [2,3]. In response to this evidence, many physical activity programs are encouraged by various institutions [4] and extensive research is being conducted by and aimed at public health professionals [5–7]. Maintaining fitness capacity (e.g., strength, endurance, agility, and balance) is a key factor in preserving mobility and independence for quotidian activity in later years.

Moreover, research demonstrated that regular physical activity is the only intervention that consistently improves functional health, maintains the energy balance and reduces the risk of lifestyle-related diseases, such as cardiometabolic diseases, obesity, and cerebrovascular diseases [8,9]. Physical activity is also effective in mitigating characteristic diseases such as sarcopenia, restoring physical strength, as well as preventing and delaying the development of disabilities [9]. On the contrary, physical inactivity is clearly related to muscle mass and strength loss: increased physical activity levels should have protective effects as a preventive measure and other lifestyle factors, such as a diet [8,9].

Among the different physical activities recommended for the elderly, Tai Chi is worth studying: Tai Chi is a traditional martial art practiced for defense and health benefits in Chinese society. In Tai Chi, which is a balance-based exercise, slow and rhythmic movements together in a continuous sequence are performed, and the center of gravity

(COG) moves with the movements of each foot. Evidence has shown many health benefits of Tai Chi [10], such as relieving psychobiological stress reactivity, promoting psychological wellbeing [11], lowering blood pressure [12], improving flexibility and muscle strength [10], and delaying the results of several chronic diseases [10,13]. The practice of Tai Chi involves lower limb control, lower limb strengthening, and dynamic posture control. People who practice Tai Chi maintain different postures and keep the COG within a changing support base to challenge their balance control system [14].

Another activity offered for this age group is Keep-Fit exercise, referring to a physical and sports activity characterised by low-impact exercises, thus without sudden and fast movements. Muscle workouts are complemented with flexibility, coordination or posture correction [15]. Keep-fit exercise considers the body as a whole: all body parts are equally important, and merge strength, endurance, and joint health. These programmes are focused on health improvements through individualised, safe and motivating exercise aimed at enhancing adherence [16–19]; the rhythm and expressive components showed differential compliance among women and men [20]: specifically, it seems that women participate in these type of activities to a greater proportion compared to males [20–22].

The effects of specific physical exercise programs on older adults have been analysed, but few studies have analysed differences in fitness capacities between different types of fitness programs [23,24]. Studying differences between programs—including its subjectively perceived attractiveness and adherence capacity—may help us to identify or design the most appropriate modalities for older adults and the ones that offer them the most significant benefits. This study aims to (a) compare and assess the functional capacity of older adults who perform supervised activities and a sedentary group (sedentary individuals versus individuals who practise Tai Chi or Keep-Fit exercise), and (b) compare the influence of a recurrent Tai Chi practice in older Chinese adults with an amateur practice of this martial art in the Spanish population.

2. Materials and Methods

2.1. Participants and Procedures

A cross-sectional descriptive biometric observational study was conducted. The physical condition evaluation was conducted through five Senior Fitness Tests (SFT) in a group of Spanish and Chinese individuals aged 65 or older. The study was designed according to the guidelines of the Declaration of Helsinki, and approved by the Institutional Review Board (or Ethics Committee) of León University (ETICA-ULE-004-2021).

In total, 113 participants (71.53 ± 6.92 years old) were divided into 3 physical activity groups and 1 sedentary control group. Of the Spanish individuals who participate in activities for older adults organised by different city councils, 36 were practising Keep-Fit exercise (KF) (n = 30 women and n = 6 men), and 27 were practising Tai Chi (TC) (n = 21 women and n = 6 men), with an average weekly practice of ±3 h over ±4 years, all of them residents in Spain. In total, 27 Chinese residents participants were considered Professional Tai Chi (PTC) athletes due to recurrently practising this sport as a lifestyle with a weekly training of ±12 h and Asian athletes competing in the Senior category (n = 12 women and n = 15 men). Twenty-three participants corresponded to the sedentary control group (SI) (n = 14 women and n = 9 men), who were not currently practising or had not practised any physical activity in recent years. (Table 1).

All subjects were informed at a meeting in their town about the evaluation of the study, its procedure, and the records and tests to perform. SFT tests were applied to all participants after the initial warm-up, thus before starting their physical activity, to avoid the effect of fatigue and differences in each group due to their different exercises. Before the competition began, the Asian groups were analysed in a regional championship in Shanghai (China). Vice Dean Ph.D. Zhu Dong of the Shanghai Sports University provided the corresponding license to intervene in this event. The other group was analysed in a senior category exhibition in Shanghai (China). Master Qingquan Fu (6th Generation Master of the Yang style taijiquan and the President of the World Yong Nian Tai Chi

Federation) provided the corresponding license to intervene in this event. All participants signed informed consent.

Table 1. Sample size and distribution in the studies and analyses carried out.

Type of Activity	Women	%	Men	%	No. of Individuals	% of Individuals
Keep-Fit exercise (KF)	30	38.96	6	16.67	36	31.86
Tai Chi (TC)	21	27.27	6	16.67	27	23.89
Professional Tai Chi (PTC)	12	15.58	15	41.67	27	23.89
Sedentary Individuals (SI)	14	18.18	9	25.00	23	20.35
Total	77		36		113	

Table 2 shows the characteristics of the exercise programmes performed by the three intervention groups. Keep Fit included a 60-min session with exercises consisting of strength, coordination and agility. The Tai Chi group also performed the routine for 1 h: the first part consisted of structural and postural control, essential positioning and equilibrium; the second part included standardised and characteristic forms; lastly, a flexibility and mobility part was included. The Chinese group, practising long-life professional Tai Chi, divided the activity during the whole day: 60 min in the morning with movements and meditation; 60 min before lunchtime including essential exercise; and a non-predefined time lapse at the end of the day focused on specific forms and flexibility.

Table 2. Characteristics of programs developed by the three active groups.

	KF	TC	PTC
Hours training per week	±3	±3	±10
Training days per week	±3	±3	±10
Years of practice	±4	±4	Lifetime
Characteristics of physical exercise programs	-Warm up -Upper and lower body strength -Agility and aerobic endurance	-Basic TC exercises -Body structure -Static and dynamic balance -Postural strength and control -Form training -Upper and lower body flexibility	-Morning chikung -Half day session: basic TC exercises, body structure, static and dynamic balance, postural strength and control -Afternoon session: forms training, upper and lower body flexibility

Where KF = Keep-Fit exercise, TC = Tai Chi, PTC = Professional Tai Chi.

2.2. Exclusion and Inclusion Criteria

Inclusion criteria were: being 65 years old or older, participating in supervised classes (Keep-Fit exercise or Tai Chi) over 4 years prior to the study or not practising any kind of physical activity regarding the group considered sedentary. The exclusion criterion applied to those who suffered any severe illness or ailment which hinders mobility.

2.3. Senior Fitness Test (SFT)

The Senior Fitness Test (SFT) is a battery of seven tests whose purpose is the functional assessment of the physical capacity of the elderly [25]. This evidence-based and validated test has been rectified to evaluate these parameters: upper and lower body strength, upper and lower body flexibility, dynamic balance, agility and aerobic endurance.

The tests carried out consisted of the 30-s chair stand and 30-s arm curl, tests for upper and lower extremity muscle strength, the back scratch and chair sit-and-reach tests for upper and lower body flexibility and the up-and-go test for agility and balance.

2.4. Statistical Analysis

The corresponding tests were applied using the statistical software IMB SPSS Statistics 25. The Student's t-test was applied for independent samples to analyse gender and nationality differences. In order to analyse the mean differences of the SFT tests, the ANOVA statistical analysis of a factor was conducted if normal standards were met in all groups. The Kruskal–Wallis test was used if normal standards were not met within the group.

Regarding post-hoc tests, in the case of the ANOVA's, the homoscedasticity assumption was not met in all cases, so Welch's statistical test was calculated. Therefore, the Games Howel statistical test was used as post-hoc testing. The Mann–Whitney U test was used for non-parametric post hoc tests. The values were expressed as mean (SD), and $p < 0.05$ was considered statistically relevant.

3. Results

Table 3 shows the anthropometric characteristics of the Spanish sample: a significantly higher BMI—in particular, for women—was observed.

Table 3. Anthropometric differences in Spanish individuals according to gender.

Anthropometric Data	Women	Men
Age (years)	72.51 ± 7.43	71.52 ± 7.74
Weight (kg)	65.96 ± 11.78	74.40 ± 8.06
Height (cm)	157.39 ± 6.51	169.07 ± 4.21
BMI (kg/m^2)	26.56 ± 4.38 *	26.00 ± 2.28

Mean values ± SD. * = p = 0.05.

When comparing the Spanish sample with the Chinese sample in terms of anthropometric measures, Chinese participants' BMI was within normal weight ranges and is significantly lower than the Spanish participants. (Table 4).

Table 4. Anthropometric differences between Spanish and Chinese individuals.

Anthropometric Data	Spanish	Chinese
Age (years)	73.00 ± 7.51	67.59 ± 3.06
Weight (kg)	68.02 ± 11.53	64.68 ± 8.34
Height (cm)	160.24 ± 7.84	166.85 ± 6.49
BMI (kg/m^2)	26.42 ± 3.96 *	23.19 ± 2.30

Mean values ± SD. * = p = 0.05.

Considering the type of physical activity performed, Spanish participants practising Tai Chi have a significantly lower BMI when compared to sedentary individuals and the group that practises Keep-Fit exercise. (Table 5).

Table 5. Anthropometric differences according to the type of physical and/or sports activity.

	Age (Years)	Weight (kg)	Height (cm)	BMI (kg/m^2)
SI	78.91 ± 9.01	70.69 ± 13.16	164.30 ± 7.77	26.09 ± 4.08
KF	71.25 ± 6.01	69.94 ± 9.15	158.55 ± 8.18	27.87 ± 3.70
TC	70.30 ± 4.94	63.18 ± 11.84	159.03 ± 6.30	24.77 ± 3.60 *

Mean values ± SD. * = p < 0.05 regarding Keep-Fit exercise. Where SI = Sedentary Individuals, KF = Keep-Fit exercise and TC = Tai Chi.

Regarding the SFT tests, Table 6 shows that the participants in the study who practice Tai Chi have significantly better values in all tests when analysing the strength, flexibility of arms and legs, and agility compared to sedentary elderly. Consequently, people belonging to the Tai Chi group are in the 100th percentile in the strength and flexibility tests, while the sedentary individuals do not exceed the 50th percentile in any test.

Table 6. Differences in SFT tests according to the type of physical activity performed.

Tests	Group Activity	
30-s chair stand (rep)	Sedentary Individuals	10.13 ± 1.96
	Keep-Fit	17.17 ± 2.96 [#]
	Tai Chi	23.22 ± 3.08 [#$]
30-s arm curl (rep)	Sedentary Individuals	13.26 ± 2.92
	Keep-Fit	21.19 ± 3.45 [#]
	Tai Chi	23.48 ± 3.42 [#]
Chair sit-and-reach (cm)	Sedentary Individuals	−4.43 ± 5.88
	Keep-Fit	−1.93 ± 5.46 [¥]
	Tai Chi	2.19 ± 4.85 [#]
Back scratch (cm)	Sedentary Individuals	−2.94 ± 3.98
	Keep-Fit	−2.43 ± 5.78 [¥]
	Tai Chi	1.02 ± 4.46 [#]
Up-and-go (s)	Sedentary Individuals	7.28 ± 1.25
	Keep-Fit	4.64 ± 0.83 [#]
	Tai Chi	4.14 ± 0.46 [#]

Mean values ± SD. [#] = $p < 0.05$ regarding sedentary individuals. [$] = $p < 0.05$ regarding Keep-Fit exercise. [¥] = $p < 0.05$ regarding Tai Chi. Where rep = number of repetitions.

Thus, for the leg strength test, the two active groups, KF and TC, obtained significantly better results than sedentary individuals. The results of those who practice Tai Chi exceed the ones of the KF group, achieving a mean of 23.22 ± 3.08 rep (100th percentile) compared to the 17.17 ± 2.96 rep of the KF group (85th percentile) and the 10.13 ± 1.96 rep of the SI group (25th percentile). Similar results were obtained in the arm strength and agility tests, with values of the TC group in the 100th percentile in both tests and the KF group in the 95th percentile, much higher than the 13.26 ± 2.92 rep (40th percentile) and the 7.28 ± 1.25 s (25th percentile) achieved by the sedentary group in the two tests, respectively.

Significant differences in the TC group were observed in the flexibility tests of both legs and arms compared to the other groups (KF and SI). In the leg flexibility test, the individuals who practise Tai Chi achieve the value of 2.19 ± 4.85 cm (60th percentile) for this test compared to the −1.93 ± 5.46 cm (20th percentile) of the KF group and −4.43 ± 5.88 cm (5th percentile) of the sedentary group. Nevertheless, in the arm flexibility test, the TC group outperformed the participants of the KF and SI groups with 1.02 ± 4.46 cm (80th percentile) again compared to the −2.43 ± 5.78 cm (45th percentile) and −2.94 ± 3.98 cm (40th percentile) achieved by these groups, respectively.

Table 7 shows the comparison of the different SFT variables studied between the two groups practising Tai Chi (amateurs vs. professionals/Spanish vs. Chinese individuals). Both groups have percentiles above 60 in all tests whilst the Chinese people group showed the most optimal values, having the 100th percentile in all tests. The main difference is observed in flexibility tests between Spanish and Chinese. Chinese individuals obtained a leg flexibility mean of 13.07 ± 3.99 cm (100th percentile) compared to 2.19 ± 4.85 cm (60th percentile) achieved by Spanish individuals and a mean of 5.48 ± 3.50 cm (100th percentile) in the arm flexibility test compared to 1.02 ± 4.46 cm (80th percentile) achieved by Spanish individuals. Strictly considering the statistics, Asian participants also outperformed in the strength tests: (a) Asian participants achieved a mean of 30.22 ± 4.36 rep (100th percentile) in the arm strength test, compared to the 23.48 ± 3.42 rep (100th percentile) achieved by the Spanish older adult; and (b) Asian participants achieved 27.70 ± 4.98 rep (100th percentile) in the leg strength test compared to 23.22 ± 3.08 rep (100th percentile) obtained by Spanish participants.

Table 7. Influence of professional vs. amateur Tai Chi practice on SFT tests.

Tests		Mean Values ± SD
30-s chair stand (rep)	Spanish	23.22 ± 3.08
	Chinese	27.70 ± 4.98 ¥
30-s arm curl (rep)	Spanish	23.48 ± 3.42
	Chinese	30.22 ± 4.36 ¥
Chair sit-and-reach (cm)	Spanish	2.19 ± 4.85
	Chinese	13.07 ± 4.00 ¥
Back scratch (cm)	Spanish	1.02 ± 4.46
	Chinese	5.48 ± 3.51 ¥
Up-and-go (s)	Spanish	4.14 ± 0.46
	Chinese	3.91 ± 0.33

Mean values ± SD. Differences in Spanish vs. Chinese individuals: ¥ = $p < 0.05$. Where rep = number of repetitions.

Men and women were compared considering physical activities and absolute values and percentiles. Both men and women who belong to the PTC group have better results in all SFT tests than sedentary individuals and those who practice Keep-Fit exercise and those with an amateur Tai Chi practice (Table 8). Furthermore, although there are significant differences between men and women in this group, all of them fall in the 100th percentile.

Table 8. Mean values in percentiles of the different physical activities and the sedentary group for SFT tests.

SFT Tests		Mean Value (Percentile)			
		SI	KF	TC	PTC
30-s chair stand (rep)	♂	10.56 ± 1.81 (20)	19.83 ± 2.85 * (85)	20.83 ± 1.72 * (100)	28.40 ± 4.48 *ab (100)
	♀	9.86 ± 2.07 (15)	16.63 ± 2.72 * (80)	23.90 ± 3.06 *a (100)	26.83 ± 5.62 *a (100)
30-s arm curl (rep)	♂	13.56 ± 1.33 (25)	21.67 ± 3.93 * (85)	22.67 ± 3.72 * (85)	31.20 ± 3.00 *ab (100)
	♀	13.07 ± 3.64 (40)	21.10 ± 3.40 * (95)	23.71 ± 3.39 * (100)	29.00 ± 5.52 *ab# (100)
Chair sit-and-reach (cm)	♂	−6.88 ± 5.23 (10)	−5.83 ± 6.67 (10)	−4.33 ± 4.88 (25)	12.73 ± 4.02 *ab (100)
	♀	−2.85 ± 5.90 (15)	−1.15 ± 4.94 (25)	4.04 ± 2.87 *a (75)	13.50 ± 4.09 *ab (100)
Back scratch (cm)	♂	−4.84 ± 4.19 (55)	−5.08 ± 4.86 (45)	−4.91 ± 3.77 (55)	6.26 ± 3.75 *ab (100)
	♀	−1.72 ± 3.44 (50)	−1.90 ± 5.87 (50)	2.71 ± 2.95 *a (80)	4.50 ± 3.03 *a (95)
Up-and-go (s)	♂	6.51 ± 1.31 (25)	4.31 ± 1.10 * (80)	4.28 ± 0.46 * (80)	4.02 ± 0.21 * (85)
	♀	7.77 ± 0.96 (15)	4.70 ± 0.77 * (80)	4.10 ± 0.45 *a (90)	3.76 ± 0.39 *a# (95)

Mean values ± SD. * = $p < 0.05$ regarding sedentary individuals. a = $p < 0.05$ regarding Keep-Fit exercise. b = $p < 0.05$ regarding Tai Chi. # = $p < 0.05$ gender differences according type of activity. Where SI = Sedentary Individuals, KF = Keep-Fit exercise, TC = Tai Chi, PTC = Professional Tai Chi and rep = number of repetitions.

No significant differences were found between men and women in the Spanish sedentary group. It should be noted that except in the arm flexibility test, the group is below the 50th percentile in all tests. Likewise, there are no significant differences between men and women in the KF and TC groups, whilst individuals practising Tai Chi had higher percentiles than those in the KF group.

Finally, Table 8 also shows how physical activity practice improved the functional capacities in both men and women regarding sedentary individuals being the continuous practice is the most critical factor concerning those capacities. Thus, to practice Tai Chi for 3 h a week—especially in women—significantly improved leg strength, arm and leg flexibility, and agility.

4. Discussion

The novelty of the present research relies on its capacity for unveiling the potential of the Tai Chi practice and long-life physical exercise in terms of functional health, adherence, enjoyment and motivation specifically aimed at seniors.

Research shows that seniors over 70 years of age practising Tai Chi, individualised balance training and exercise control education report an overall improvement in their quotidian activities and their lives in general. In addition, subjects reported greater confidence in balance and movement and changed their usual physical activity to incorporate the continuous practice of TC [26].

Compared to no intervention or other exercises, the present study found that Tai Chi can significantly improve functional mobility and balance in the Tai Chi groups compared to the other groups that received no intervention or other active therapies. Data suggest that when mental and physical control is perceived to be enhanced, with a generalised sense of improvement in overall wellbeing, older persons' motivation to continue exercising also increases. Diverse research highlighted the TC effects on physical fitness, wellbeing, and general cognition in older adults who practice Tai Chi [27]. Moreover, research showed a psychoemotional outcome related to the development of positive emotions results as well as the emotional connections established in the practice of this martial art [28].

When comparing the group of Spanish individuals who practised Tai Chi or KF with the sedentary group, those practising Tai Chi achieved significantly better results for all SFT tests conducted. In particular, those practising Tai Chi achieved better results: (a) compared to the sedentary individuals; and (b) compared to the results achieved by the KF individuals in leg strength tests and the two flexibility tests. Additionally, those individuals practising KF outperformed the Sedentary Individuals in the two strength and agility tests. Therefore, accordingly to the current research and the literature, these assessed activities would positively affect the performance of basic tasks by the elderly—e.g., sitting down and getting up from a chair or climbing stairs, optimising typical self-care flection movements and the ability to function independently [29]. When comparing these results with similar studies for both genders, older adults who spend more than 4 h a day sitting down (Sedentary Individuals) have worse results in balance, agility, walking speed, strength and aerobic endurance tests [30–32]. The improved muscle strength among the participants in the interventions groups is gripping, considering that muscle strength naturally may decline with age. Maintenance of muscle strength may prevent loss of functional dependence [33]. A systematic review reported that exercise might prevent falls and fall-related fractures and reduce risk factors for falls in individuals with low bone mineral density [33].

The current research demonstrated that individuals practising Tai Chi have a better physical condition than those who practised KF or were sedentary. These results are aligned with the literature: significant improvements were obtained in static and dynamic balance, flexibility, and lower and upper body strength tests, as well as improvements in cardiovascular endurance with a Tai Chi practice intervention [34]. Different non-randomised controlled studies and observational studies also assessed this martial art to treat body balance disorder or fall prevention, suggesting that its practice may improve body balance in older people [35] and an added increase in cognitive function [36]. These findings indicate that a short-term and intensive physical training program improves the lower body physical function: for instance, dynamic balance and leg strength and enhances the upper body physical function, fine motor control, and strength [37,38]. These data are also higher for the individuals practising Keep-Fit exercise, as seen in other studies [39], proving that this activity also improves the physical condition in older people when comparing them with sedentary people. Still, our study demonstrated an enhanced physical condition due to practising Tai Chi compared to KF.

Nevertheless, there are differences in our study group when compared with the results obtained in similar samples. Another study [40] including a sample of Spanish people over 80 was compared with the American SFT reference values: better strength and agility results and lower flexibility and resistance levels were observed in the Spanish individuals than in the reference American population, not showing significant differences between genders in the Spanish population. In turn, this fact can also be observed in the study conducted [41] between Spanish and Serbian older women who practised different physical activities: Serbian women showed better physical fitness, upper and lower body flexibility, agility and aerobic endurance, i.e., better levels of physical condition and quality of life than the Spanish women, differences attributed to the type of physical activity performed by both groups.

Consistent physical training improves all aspects studied regardless of the participant's age: the present research shows how older people who have practised Tai Chi almost all their lives and who, at the time of our study, were training for more than 10 h a week, have a significantly higher physical capacity in all physical characteristics studied.

Similar research studying eventual differences in physical fitness and health in Asian and European older adults shows significantly higher performance levels in motor skills—i.e., aerobic fitness, strength and flexibility—for the Asian sample, aligned the significantly higher results achieved by Chinese individuals in the strength and flexibility tests conducted in our study [42]. Other authors [43] revealed similar differences by observing a consistently lower incidence of self-reported falls in Chinese older people than in Caucasian older people [44,45]. Therefore, a greater understanding of the health, behavioural and lifestyle factors that influence fall rates in Chinese populations is required to elucidate fall prevention strategies in older people. Older Chinese people frequently perform physical activities with low and medium intensity, and maintaining an active lifestyle is a characteristic of this population thus the better physical fitness of the Chinese group assessed in our study may be related to practising Tai Chi throughout their lives [46].

Along these lines, policies aimed at promoting physical exercise and sports throughout the whole lifecycle are needed in order to reduce the impact of the ageing process in modern occidental societies and lessen the health inequalities caused by the lack of access to sports facilities for the most vulnerable populations [47,48]. Our research suggests that Tai Chi and other non-conventional sports and martial arts can be adapted and delivered to senior and older populations and the whole society, offering an attractive and effective alternative in terms of healthy ageing, functional health and socialization [49,50].

5. Limitations and Future Research Lines

The present research showed an analysis of the physical condition and functionality of one of the most offered activities aimed at older persons, the Keep Fit, compared, as a feasible alternative, with Tai Chi. The innovation of the study relies on the possibility of studying the effects of a different lifestyle—i.e., the Chinese population—and the long-life and continued physical activity, introducing an international sample of Chinese subjects practising TC. The potential influence of the ethnicity and ethnic factors should be further studied and will be assessed in future research. Considering that the present research compares groups with very different profiles—i.e., Tai Chi professionals, older people who exercise regularly, or sedentary persons—it is recommended for future research to keep track of each training and quality of life of each sample. Whilst the improvement of health indicators with the practice of physical activity and specifically of physical condition with Tai Chi seems to be demonstrated. It is also considered necessary to address the exercise recommendations for this population considering the structural co-determinants: spaces, infrastructures, affordability and opportunities to socialise, enjoy and feel heard and seem should be integrated within the general research and the public health programmes.

6. Conclusions

The present research shows how the practice of a physical activity aimed at older persons significantly improves their physical condition. The practice of Tai Chi stands out as physical activity compared to Keep-Fit or physical inactivity, significantly improving physical condition for this age group. Considering the variety of physical activities recommended for seniors, Tai Chi outperforms Keep-Fit in the results, particularly within the SFT tests outcomes. Specifically, long-life training of Tai Chi—as it is being practised among the Chinese population—shows even more significant improvements in leg and arm strength, upper and lower body flexibility, and agility. Our study reviewed effects on seniors' wellbeing and general cognition and the development of positive emotions with the practice of Tai Chi. Therefore, there is a need to generate policies and strategies for promoting sports and physical activity to reduce the ageing, adverse health and functionality consequences, considering and tackling the structural co-determinants involved.

Author Contributions: All authors actively contributed to the present research paper: conceptualization and methodology, A.N.; software and validation, P.S.C.; formal analysis and investigation, A.N.; resources and data curation, J.G.V.-V.; writing—original draft preparation, A.N.; writing—review and editing, P.S.C. and J.G.V.-V.; visualization and supervision, P.S.C. and J.G.V.-V. All authors have read and agreed to the published version of the manuscript.

Funding: This research received no external funding.

Institutional Review Board Statement: The study was conducted according to the guidelines of the Declaration of Helsinki and approved by the Institutional Review Board (or Ethics Committee) of León University (ETICA-ULE-004-2021).

Informed Consent Statement: Informed consent was obtained from all subjects involved in the study. The patient(s) has obtained written informed consent to publish this paper.

Data Availability Statement: Not Applicable.

Acknowledgments: The collaboration of the Shanghai Sports University (China) and the license of Vice Dean Zhu Dong and Master Qingquan Fu (6th Generation Master of the Yang style taijiquan and the President of the Word Yong Nian Tai Chi Federation) to intervene in the samples of the Chinese population of the elderly are appreciated. Also, thank the Tai Chi clubs for their participation in the study, the volunteers and the Asturian Federation of Judo and Associated Sports (FAJYDA) and the Royal Spanish Federation of Judo and Associated Sports (RFEJYDA).

Conflicts of Interest: Authors have no conflict of interest, and the results of the study are presented clearly, honestly, and without fabrication, falsification, or inappropriate data manipulation.

References

1. Silva, F.M.; Petrica, J.; Serrano, J.; Paulo, R.; Ramalho, A.; Lucas, D.; Ferreira, J.P.; Duarte-Mendes, P. The sedentary time and physical activity levels on physical fitness in the elderly: A comparative cross sectional study. *Int. J. Environ. Res. Public Health* **2019**, *16*, 3697. [CrossRef]
2. Ngandu, T.; Lehtisalo, J.; Solomon, A.; Levälahti, E.; Ahtiluoto, S.; Antikainen, R.; Bäckman, L.; Hänninen, T.; Jula, A.; Laatikainen, T.; et al. A 2 year multidomain intervention of diet, exercise, cognitive training, and vascular risk monitoring versus control to prevent cognitive decline in at-risk elderly people (FINGER): A randomised controlled trial. *Lancet* **2015**, *385*, 2255–2263. [CrossRef]
3. Rosenberg, D.; Cook, A.J.; Gell, N.; Lozano, P.; Grothaus, L.; Arterburn, D. Relationships between sitting time and health indicators, costs, and utilization in older adults. *Prev. Med. Rep.* **2015**, *2*, 247–249. [CrossRef]
4. Heath, G.W.; Parra, D.C.; Sarmiento, O.L.; Andersen, L.B.; Owen, N.; Goenka, S.; Montes, F.; Brownson, R.C.; for the Lancet Physical Activity Series Working Group. Evidence-based intervention in physical activity: Lessons from around the world. *Lancet* **2012**, *380*, 272–281. [CrossRef]
5. Greaves, C.J.; Sheppard, K.E.; Abraham, C.; Hardeman, W.; Roden, M.; Evans, P.H.; Schwarz, P. The IMAGE Study Group. Systematic review of reviews of intervention components associated with increased effectiveness in dietary and physical activity interventions. *BMC Public Health* **2011**, *11*, 119. [CrossRef] [PubMed]
6. Kohl, H.W., 3rd; Craig, C.L.; Lambert, E.V.; Inoue, S.; Alkandari, J.R.; Leetongin, G.; Kahlmeier, S. Lancet Physical Activity Series Working Group. The pandemic of physical inactivity: Global action for public health. *Lancet* **2012**, *380*, 294–305. [CrossRef]
7. Rondanelli, M.; Klersy, C.; Terracol, G.; Talluri, J.; Maugeri, R.; Guido, D.; Faliva, M.A.; Solerte, B.S.; Fioravanti, M.; Lukaski, H.; et al. Whey protein, amino acids, and vitamin D supplementation with physical activity increases fat-free mass and strength, functionality, and quality of life and decreases inflammation in sarcopenic elderly. *Am. J. Clin. Nutr.* **2016**, *103*, 830–840. [CrossRef]
8. Izquierdo, M.; Merchant, R.A.; Morley, J.E.; Anker, S.D.; Aprahamian, I.; Arai, H.; Aubertin-Leheudre, M.; Bernabei, R.; Cadore, E.L.; Cesari, M.; et al. International Exercise Recommendations in Older Adults (ICFSR): Expert Consensus Guidelines. *J. Nutr. Health Aging* **2021**, *25*, 824–853. [CrossRef]

9. Marzetti, E.; Calvani, R.; Tosato, M.; Cesari, M.; Di Bari, M.; Cherubini, A.; Broccatelli, M.; Savera, G.; D'Elia, M.; Pahor, M.; et al. Physical activity and exercise as countermeasures to physical frailty and sarcopenia. *Aging Clin. Exp. Res.* **2017**, *29*, 35–42. [CrossRef]
10. Lan, C.; Lai, J.-S.; Chen, S.-Y.; Wong, A.M.-K. 12-month Tai Chi training in the elderly: Its effect on health fitness. *Med. Sci. Sports Exerc.* **1998**, *30*, 345–351. [CrossRef]
11. Wang, F.; Lee, E.K.O.; Wu, T.; Benson, H.; Fricchione, G.; Wang, W.; Yeung, A.S. The effects of tai chi on depression, anxiety, and psychological wellbeing: A systematic review and meta-analysis. *Int. J. Behav. Med.* **2014**, *21*, 605–617. [CrossRef] [PubMed]
12. Yeh, G.Y.; Wang, C.; Wayne, P.M.; Phillips, R.S. The effect of tai chi exercise on blood pressure: A systematic review. *Prev. Cardiol.* **2008**, *11*, 82–89. [CrossRef] [PubMed]
13. Wang, C.; Schmid, C.H.; Fielding, R.A.; Harvey, W.F.; Reid, K.F.; Price, L.L.; Driban, J.B.; Kalish, R.; Rones, R.; McAlindon, T. Effect of tai chi versus aerobic exercise for fibromyalgia: Comparative effectiveness randomised controlled trial. *Br. Med. J.* **2018**, *360*, k851. [CrossRef] [PubMed]
14. Huang, Y.; Liu, X. Improvement of balance control ability and flexibility in the elderly Tai Chi Chuan (TCC) practitioners: A systematic review and meta-analysis. *Arch. Gerontol. Geriatr.* **2015**, *60*, 233–238. [CrossRef]
15. Moreno, J.A.; Marín de Oliveira, L.M. Análisis de los motivos de práctica entre usuarios de programas tradicionales y de fitness. In *Actas del Congreso Internacional de Actividades Acuáticas*; Universidad de Murcia: Murcia, Spain, 2003; pp. 26–28.
16. Meredith, M.D. Activity or fitness: Is the process or the product more important for public health? *Quest* **1988**, *40*, 180–186. [CrossRef]
17. Jetté, M.; Quenneville, J.; Sidney, K. Fitness Testing and Counselling in Health Promotion. *Can. J. Sport Sci.* **1995**, *17*, 194–198.
18. Mahoney, C. Health Related Exercise in Northern Ireland. *Bull. Phys. Educ.* **1993**, *29*, 21–24.
19. Morrow, J.R.; Gill, D.L. Physical Activity, Fitness, and Health: Introduction. *Quest* **1995**, *47*, 261–262. [CrossRef]
20. Macías, V.; Moya, M. Género y Deporte. La influencia de las variables psicosociales sobre la práctica deportiva de jóvenes de ambos sexos. *Rev. Psicol. Soc.* **2002**, *17*, 129–148. [CrossRef]
21. Aguila Soto, C.; Sicilia, A.; Muyor, J.M.; Orta Cantón, A. Cultura posmoderna y perfiles de práctica en los centros deportivos municipales. *Rev. Int. Med. Cienc. Act. Fís. Deporte* **2009**, *9*, 81–95.
22. López-Cozar, R.; Rebollo, S. Análisis de la relación entre práctica deportiva y características sociodemográficas en personas mayores. *Rev. Int. Med. Cienc. Act. Fís. Deporte* **2002**, *2*, 69–98.
23. Viladrosa, M.; Lavedán, A.; Jürschik, P.; Mas-Alòs, S.; Anzano, A.P.; Masot, O. Differences in fitness level between women aged 60 and over participating in three different supervised exercise programs and a sedentary group. *J. Women Aging* **2018**, *30*, 326–343. [CrossRef] [PubMed]
24. Bullo, V.; Bergamin, M.; Gobbo, S.; Sieverdes, J.C.; Zaccaria, M.; Neunhaeuserer, D.; Ermolao, A. The effects of Pilates exercise training on physical fitness and wellbeing in the elderly: A systematic review for future exercise prescription. *Prev. Med.* **2015**, *75*, 1–11. [CrossRef]
25. Jones, C.J.; Rikli, R.E. Measuring functional. *J. Act. Aging* **2002**, *1*, 24–30.
26. Kutner, N.G.; Barnhart, H.; Wolf, S.L.; McNeely, E.; Xu, T. Self-report benefits of Tai Chi practice by older adults. *J. Gerontol. Ser. B Psychol. Sci. Soc. Sci.* **1997**, *52*, P242–P246. [CrossRef]
27. Kim, T.H.M.; Pascual-Leone, J.; Johnson, J.; Tamim, H. The mental-attention Tai Chi effect with older adults. *BMC Psychol.* **2016**, *4*, 29. [CrossRef]
28. Yao, L.; Giordani, B.; Alexander, N.B. Developing a positive emotion–motivated Tai Chi (PEM-TC) exercise program for older adults with dementia. *Res. Theory Nurs. Pract.* **2008**, *22*, 241–255. [CrossRef]
29. Morris, M.; Shoo, A. Optimising exercise and physical activity in older people. *Physiother. Theory Pract.* **2004**, *20*, 143. [CrossRef]
30. Purath, J.; Buchholz, S.W.; Kark, D.L. Physical fitness assessment of older adults in the primary care setting. *J. Am. Acad. Nurse Pract.* **2009**, *21*, 101–107. [CrossRef]
31. Gouveia, R.; Maia, J.A.; Beunen, G.P.; Blimkie, C.J.; Fena, E.M.; Freitas, D.L. Functional Fitness and Physical Activity of Portuguese Community-Residing Older Adults. *J. Aging Phys. Act.* **2013**, *21*, 1–19. [CrossRef]
32. Sagarra-Romero, L.; Vicente-Rodríguez, G.; Pedrero-Chamizo, R.; Vila-Maldonado, S.; Gusi, N.; Villa-Vicente, J.G.; Espino, L.; González-Gross, M.; Casajús, J.A.; Ara, I.; et al. Is sitting time related with physical fitness in Spanish elderly population? The EXERNET multicenter study. *J. Nutr. Health Aging* **2019**, *23*, 401–407. [CrossRef] [PubMed]
33. Stanghelle, B.; Bentzen, H.; Giangregorio, L.; Pripp, A.H.; Skelton, D.A.; Bergland, A. Physical fitness in older women with osteoporosis and vertebral fracture after a resistance and balance exercise programme: 3-month post-intervention follow-up of a randomised controlled trial. *BMC Musculoskelet. Disord.* **2020**, *21*, 471. [CrossRef] [PubMed]
34. Soto, J.R.; Dopico, X.; Giraldez, M.A.; Iglesias, E.; Amador, F. La incidencia de programas de actividad física en la población de adultos mayores. *Motricidad. Eur. J. Hum. Mov.* **2009**, *22*, 65–81.
35. Maciaszek, J.; Osiński, W. The effects of Tai Chi on body balance in elderly people—A review of studies from the early 21st century. *Am. J. Chin. Med.* **2010**, *38*, 219–229. [CrossRef] [PubMed]
36. Wayne, P.M.; Walsh, J.N.; Taylor-Piliae, R.E.; Wells, R.E.; Papp, K.V.; Donovan, N.J.; Yeh, G.Y. Effect of Tai Chi on cognitive performance in older adults: Systematic review and meta-analysis. *J. Am. Geriatr. Soc.* **2014**, *62*, 25–39. [CrossRef] [PubMed]
37. Hong, Y.; Li, J.X.; Robinson, P.D. Balance control, flexibility, and cardiorespiratory fitness among older Tai Chi practitioners. *Br. J. Sports Med.* **2000**, *34*, 29–34. [CrossRef]

38. Lou, L.; Zou, L.; Fang, Q.; Wang, H.; Liu, Y.; Tian, Z.; Han, Y. Effect of Taichi softball on function-related outcomes in older adults: A randomised control trial. *Evid. Based Complement. Altern. Med.* **2017**, *2017*, 4585424. [CrossRef]
39. Carral, J.M.C.; Fernández, F.C.; Pérez, V.R. Efecto de un programa de fortalecimiento muscular en un colectivo de mujeres mayores de 65 años. *Gerokomos Rev. Soc. Esp. Enferm. Geriátr. Gerontol.* **2003**, *14*, 80–89.
40. Sanz, A.N.; Galache, A.G.; Ureña, R.M.; Montes, C.N.; Sedano, L.R.; López, A.M.; de la Rosa, Á.P.; Leiva, H.M. Valoración de la condición física mediante el senior fitness test y el índice de masa corporal en una muestra española de personas mayores de 80 años. *Arch. Med. Deporte* **2019**, *36*, 232–236.
41. Ruiz-Montero, P.J.; Castillo-Rodríguez, A.; Mikalački, M.; Delgado-Fernández, M. Physical Fitness Comparison and Quality of Life between Spanish and Serbian Elderly Women through a Physical Fitness Program. *Coll. Antropol.* **2015**, *39*, 411–417.
42. Nguyen, H.M.; Cihlar, V. Differences in Physical Fitness and Subjectively Rated Physical Health in Vietnamese and German Older Adults. *J. Cross-Cult. Gerontol.* **2013**, *28*, 181–194. [CrossRef] [PubMed]
43. Kwan, M.M.-S.; Close, J.C.; Wong, A.K.W.; Lord, S.R. Falls Incidence, Risk Factors, and Consequences in Chinese Older People: A Systematic Review. *J. Am. Geriatr. Soc.* **2011**, *59*, 536–543. [CrossRef]
44. Huang, Z.; Feng, Y.-H.; Li, Y.-H.; Lv, C.-S. Systematic review and meta-analysis: Tai Chi for preventing falls in older adults. *BMJ Open* **2017**, *7*, e013661. [CrossRef] [PubMed]
45. Zhong, D.; Xiao, Q.; Xiao, X.; Li, Y.; Ye, J.; Xia, L.; Zhang, C.; Li, J.; Zheng, H.; Jin, R. Tai Chi for improving balance and reducing falls: An overview of 14 systematic reviews. *Ann. Phys. Rehabil. Med.* **2020**, *63*, 505–517. [CrossRef] [PubMed]
46. Wang, H. Survey of physical activity and health among Chinese senior citizens over 70 years old. *Zhonghua Yu Fang Yi Xue Za Zhi* **2015**, *49*, 1005–1008.
47. Haudenhuyse, R. The impact of austerity on poverty and sport participation: Mind the knowledge gap. *Int. J. Sport Policy Politics* **2017**, *10*, 203–213. [CrossRef]
48. Sumption, B.; Burnett, C. Live in the moment, educate for life: Lessons for life-long participation in structured physical activity. *J. Phys. Educ. Sport* **2021**, *21*, 165–173. [CrossRef]
49. Adams, K.B.; Leibbrandt, S.; Moon, H. A critical review of the literature on social and leisure activity and wellbeing in later life. *Ageing Soc.* **2011**, *31*, 683–712. [CrossRef]
50. Weiss, O.; Norden, G. Socialisation and Sport. In *Introduction to the Sociology of Sport*; Brill: Leiden, The Netherlands, 2021; pp. 52–98.

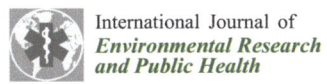

International Journal of
Environmental Research and Public Health

Article

The Acceptability of Physical Activity to Older Adults Living in Lower Socioeconomic Status Areas: A Multi-Perspective Study

Angela Devereux-Fitzgerald [1,*], Rachael Powell [2] and David P. French [2]

1. Division of Nursing, Midwifery and Social Work, School of Health Sciences, University of Manchester, Manchester M13 9PL, UK
2. Manchester Centre for Health Psychology, Division of Psychology & Mental Health, School of Health Sciences, University of Manchester, Manchester M13 9PL, UK; rachael.powell@manchester.ac.uk (R.P.); David.french@manchester.ac.uk (D.P.F.)
* Correspondence: angela.devereux@manchester.ac.uk

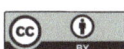

Citation: Devereux-Fitzgerald, A.; Powell, R.; French, D.P. The Acceptability of Physical Activity to Older Adults Living in Lower Socioeconomic Status Areas: A Multi-Perspective Study. *Int. J. Environ. Res. Public Health* **2021**, *18*, 11784. https://doi.org/10.3390/ijerph182211784

Academic Editors: Andy Pringle and Nicola Kime

Received: 30 September 2021
Accepted: 1 November 2021
Published: 10 November 2021

Publisher's Note: MDPI stays neutral with regard to jurisdictional claims in published maps and institutional affiliations.

Copyright: © 2021 by the authors. Licensee MDPI, Basel, Switzerland. This article is an open access article distributed under the terms and conditions of the Creative Commons Attribution (CC BY) license (https://creativecommons.org/licenses/by/4.0/).

Abstract: Older adults in lower socioeconomic status (SES) areas are the least active of all adult groups but are often absent from physical activity research. The present study aimed to elicit perspectives on acceptability of physical activity from older adults and physical activity providers in lower SES areas. Semi-structured interviews were conducted with 19 older adults and eight physical activity trainers/providers in lower SES areas. An inductive, multi-perspective Thematic Analysis was conducted. Eight themes were identified that covered one or both groups' perceptions of what was important in ensuring acceptability of activity provision. Older adults perceived a lack of value that was reinforced by lack of resources and unequal provision. Acceptability was hindered by centralisation of facilities and lack of understanding of needs by facility management. Facilitating social interaction within physical activities appeared key, thereby meeting multiple needs with fewer resources. In conclusion, to increase acceptability of physical activity for older adults in low SES areas, providers should address the lack of perceived value felt by many older adults. Equitable provision of physical activities addressing multiple needs may allow older adults with limited resources to be physically active without sacrificing other needs. Facilitating creation of social bonds may foster maintenance of physical activities.

Keywords: inequality; ageing; deprivation; physical activity; exercise; acceptability; trainers; providers; qualitative

1. Introduction

Physical activity provides multiple benefits for older adults, including lowered risk of chronic illness and mortality, maintenance of cognitive and physical function, improved mood, and increased quality of life [1,2]. However, physical activity declines with age [3], with the majority of older adults (65+ years) in England not meeting current physical activity guidelines [4]. People in the most deprived areas are twice as likely to be inactive as those in the least deprived areas [5]. Furthermore, older adults in lower socioeconomic status (SES) areas can experience greater environmental and individual barriers to engaging in leisure-time physical activity than the general older adult population [6–9]. Despite these factors, older adults in lower SES areas are often absent from qualitative studies concerning both the concept of physical activity and engagement with behaviour-change interventions to increase physical activity [10,11].

If the acceptability of behaviour change interventions is overlooked, their effectiveness may be undermined [12]. Acceptability of health behaviour interventions has generally been conceptualised as the level of tolerance required to undertake health interventions or, more recently, the perceived appropriateness to those delivering or receiving a healthcare intervention based on their cognitive and emotional responses [13]. However, physical activity differs from many health behaviours, such as screening and adherence to medication, as it may be viewed as a desirable activity of itself—a pleasurable way to spend time connecting with others or reconnecting with oneself [14]. Acceptability of physical activity is therefore a more nuanced concept, incorporating context, such as resources, setting, delivery, experience, and meaning of physical activity, in order to determine individual acceptability [10,11,15]. Hence, simply identifying older adults' motivations, beliefs, and barriers to engaging in physical activity (e.g., [16]) may pay insufficient attention to the impact of context.

Those who provide or deliver physical activity (hereafter referred to as trainers/ providers) are key aspects of this context. King [8] noted that interpersonal approaches are most effective for engaging older adults in physical activity, with an incremental, empathic approach to delivery being highly acceptable [11]. It has been suggested that perceptions of individual characteristics of trainers/providers (including attitude, age, experience, training) influence engagement at the start of a physical activity programme as well as maintenance of physical activity in the general older adult population [17,18]. However, there has been little qualitative research into the experiences of those providing physical activity to older adults in low SES areas, where greater barriers exist. For example, two recent systematic reviews of the experiences of older adults regarding physical activity found only 1 out of 17 studies included low SES adults [10,11].

To improve services and increase engagement, we need to better understand what constitutes acceptable physical activity provision for older adults. We also need to understand what those who provide and deliver physical activity services within low SES locations perceive to be acceptable to older adults. The present qualitative study therefore aimed to elicit and analyse the views of older adults living in lower SES areas around the acceptability of engaging in physical activity to better inform future provision of physical activity services within these areas. It also aimed to elicit and analyse what trainers/providers perceive to be important in ensuring acceptability of activity provision for older adults in lower SES areas. Gaining the perspectives of both groups allows different but related issues to be examined concurrently, giving greater insight to the overall phenomenon as well as triangulating the data [19].

2. Materials and Methods

2.1. Design

A multi-perspective design used semi-structured interviews to elicit views and experiences of older adults and trainers/providers in relation to the acceptability of physical activity services to older adults.

2.2. Participants

All participants were recruited from lower SES areas of Manchester, England, a city which itself is deprived relative to much of the rest of the country. Fifteen areas within the city were selected based specifically on the percentage level of deprivation that older adults in those areas experienced [20] in order to target participants living and working in the most relevant context for the study. In the eligible areas at the time of recruitment, between 38.5 per cent and 54.8 per cent of older adults were living in deprivation (compared to the national English average of 18.1 per cent), where deprivation was based on factors including crime risk, living environment, access to local amenities, and income [20].

Older adults were eligible to take part if they were aged at least 65 years, lived independently in the lower SES areas described, had sufficient English language capability for an interview, and could walk without stopping for 10 min without assistance (walking aids permissible). Trainers/providers were eligible if they were over 18 and involved in delivering physical activity classes or services to adults 65 years old and over in a paid or voluntary capacity and in any of the specified lower SES areas. Purposive sampling aimed for variation in the older adult sample in terms of activity levels, age, and residential area, and for trainers/ providers, type of sector serviced, and type of activity provided.

Service area data collection took place March–July 2015. Interviews were conducted until data saturation was reached. Initial recruitment was publicised via age-related charities, newsletters (research groups and local government), and libraries, together with a snowballing approach where further possible participants were identified by those who had already taken part. The first author visited coffee mornings, community social and craft groups, and physical activity sessions aimed at older adults to enhance recruitment, as face-to-face recruitment regarding physical activity research has been found effective in the older adult population [21]. The first author was familiar with similar low SES settings and seemed readily accepted by participants.

2.3. Procedure

Institutional ethical approval was granted. Eligibility was established and participant information sheets delivered. Informed consent (including for use of anonymized quotes) was gained prior to face-to-face interviews, which were conducted by the first author at the participant's home or work or at the first author's university. The interviews consisted of two parts: a structured questionnaire to obtain demographic and background data, immediately followed by the semi-structured interview. No financial remuneration was provided beyond travel expenses for those who attended the university. Data from previous interviews were considered throughout in an iterative process, so emerging topics could be addressed in later interviews. This process continued until data saturation became apparent. Field notes were taken after interviews to retain context. Interviews lasted 31–95 min (median 61 min) and were audio-recorded.

2.4. Materials

The structured questionnaires covered demographic questions and included items about physical activity levels and car ownership (older adults) and work role, delivery sector, and physical activity type provided (trainers/providers). Older adults' physical activity levels were established based on the amount of time (min per week) participants self-reported spending on light, moderate, or vigorous physical activities: they were denoted as highly active if they met the recommended guideline of 150 min of moderate/75 min of vigorous physical activity per week plus worked on strength building and flexibility [2], active if they met the 150 min of moderate/75 min of vigorous physical activity per week and did not report engaging in strength/flexibility activities, somewhat active if they did some moderate/vigorous physical activity per week but did not meet the guidelines, and lower activity if they did not report engaging in any physical activity beyond basic daily living.

Semi-structured interviews were facilitated by interview schedules focusing on factors of acceptability of physical activity, updated as necessary with suggested topics from ongoing interviews with both groups. The older adults' interview schedule (see Supplementary S1) included how participants felt about physical activity, their physical activity levels, physical activity likes/dislikes, benefits or concerns, and local physical activity provision. The trainers/providers' interview schedule (see Supplementary S2) included motivation for working with older adults and physical activity, what older adults wanted regarding physical activity, local physical activity provision, barriers for older adults, attendance and feedback received, and experiences of increasing older adults' physical activity engagement.

2.5. Analysis

A Thematic Analysis was conducted to examine the experiences of the participants [22], using data management principles of the Framework Approach [23]. This encouraged breadth and depth in the exploration of the data by the research team whilst facilitating transparent and accessible data management and a clear audit trail. The analysis was conducted from a critical realist perspective; we sought the views and perceptions of participants in multiple contexts to expand our understanding of the reality of the topic at hand (e.g., [24]). Interviews were transcribed verbatim, read repeatedly to achieve familiarisation, and topics relevant to the research question were identified. Initial codes were generated from both groups' data concurrently and collated into a single hierarchical coding framework of potential themes and sub-themes. Both explicit and latent themes were explored by the whole research team, thereby incorporating the different work and life experiences the team members brought to the study. Such experience included various levels of previous work with older adults, with physical activity, and with qualitative research. Additionally, the first author's interest in this work was initially fuelled by her own experience of growing up, living, and working in low SES areas and driven forward by the powerful interactions with the participants themselves. In line with the Framework approach, matrices were produced in Excel to facilitate thematic and case-based analysis, with themes discussed and merged or split as necessary. The matrices assisted the analysis through identification of patterns within the data, identifying links between same or different phenomena and any notable absence of such links [25]. Final themes were elicited from analysis of such patterns and the interconnected nature of the themes (see Figure 1 for a thematic overview). Concurrent analysis allowed for a deeper exploration of each theme from a multi-perspective stance and allowed cross-case analysis to also highlight differences and similarities in perspectives.

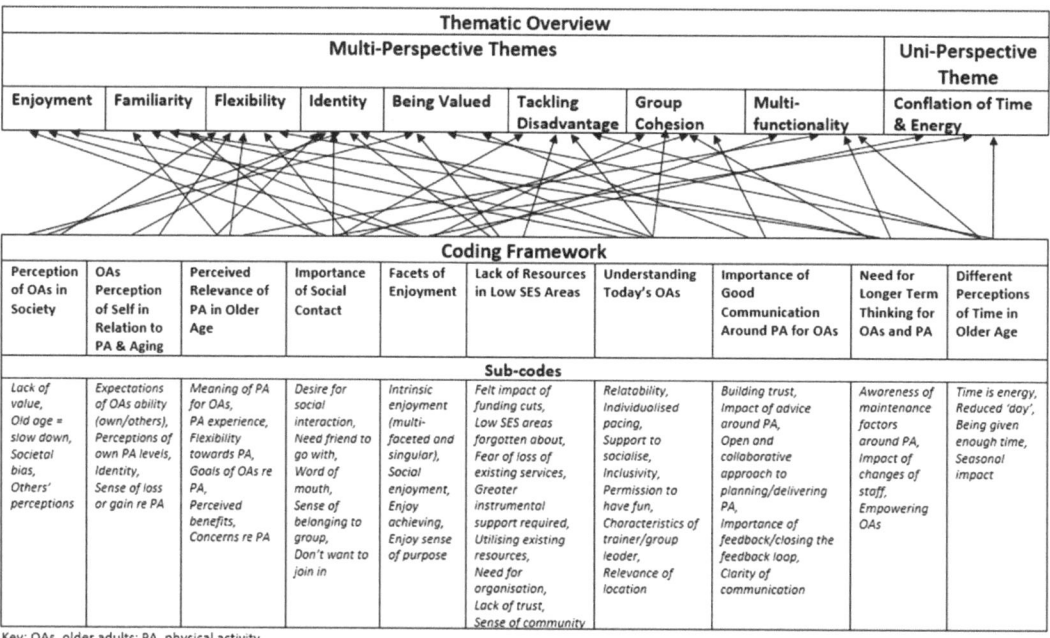

Figure 1. Thematic overview showing relationship between themes and coding framework.

3. Results

Table 1 below shows sociodemographic data for all participants. Of the 19 older adult participants, four identified as White Irish, one as British Pakistani, and 14 as White British. Two married couples participated and were interviewed individually. Ten older adults lived alone, 7 lived with their spouse, and two lived with other family members. Four participants across three households had access to a car. Participants were categorized as being highly active ($n = 6$), active ($n = 3$), somewhat active ($n = 3$), or low activity ($n = 7$) based on self-reported physical activity.

Table 1. Sociodemographic Characteristics of Participants.

Sociodemographic Characteristic	Older Adults n = 19 Age in Years 67–94 (M = 74.4, SD = 7.1)		Trainers/Providers n = 8 Age in Years 30–62 (M = 43.5, SD = 12.5)	
	n	%	n	%
Gender				
Female	15	79	5	62.5
Male	4	21	3	37.5
Marital Status				
Married	7	36.8		
Widowed	6	31.6	Not reported	Not reported
Divorced	3	15.8		
Single	3	15.8		
Education				
Did not complete secondary education	5	26.3		
Completed secondary education	7	36.8	Not reported	Not reported
Further education	5	26.3		
PhD	2	10.5		

Of the eight trainer/provider participants, one was a volunteer, and the rest held paid positions. Most trainers/providers (n = 6) identified as White British (detailed breakdown not provided to protect participant identity due to the relatively small participant pool). Length of time working in physical activity for older adults ranged from 0.5 to 15 years (M = 5.64, SD = 4.73). The physical activities they offered included walking, Tai Chi, circuit training, dancing, walking football, and seated exercises.

The thematic analysis produced eight themes: being valued, tackling disadvantage, flexibility, familiarity, enjoyment, identity, group cohesion, and multi-functionality. A further theme explaining differences in perception of time in older age was found in the older adult sample alone and is discussed in detail in a separate publication [26]. Pseudonyms have been used for all quotes to preserve anonymity of participants. Gender, age, and activity levels are noted for older adults, and gender, age, and role are noted for trainer/providers.

3.1. Being Valued

A general lack of value of older adults in society was perceived:

This world isn't built for old people [. . .] nobody respects you [. . .] You're given no respect for what you've done. You know, it's . . . I don't know. I think it's very sad because we've got a lot that we could share with young people. But it's got to be a two-way thing. You know, they've got to build us in when, you know, these people with budgets. They've got to build us into that as well. You know, we've got to be brought into the equation and then we've got a lot to share. (Linda, F, 68, Low activity)

This lack of value seemed exacerbated in low SES areas, where physical activities were often provided in shared community facilities rather than the dedicated spaces available in higher SES areas (e.g., tennis/golf clubs). There was a perception that older adults' low-revenue activities were more prone to cancellation than others in shared facilities: *"Every time that the pool is needed, it's always the [older adults' aquafit] that get told 'Your exercise is cancelled'"* (Kevin, M, 71, Highly active). Some trainer/providers tried to show older adults that they were valued: *"Talk to them, ask them how their day's been. Ask them where they're going after this. [. . .] Listen to what they've got to say"* (James, M, 30, Trainer). Being offered something perceived as being desirable to others, knowledge of substantial discounts, or brand recognition increased acceptability:

Zumba's really popular, and that's popular because it's quite expensive normally to pay for if you were just to go into a gym or whatever. So, when we put those on locally, they're received well. Cos it's something that they have heard about. (Emma, F, 33, Provider)

Lack of funding led to lack of marketing, resulting in some older adults perceiving being overlooked in favour of other groups: *"I've never seen an advert about senior citizens swimming—there's plenty of things about, you know, youngsters, school children, that sort of thing"* (Pam, F, 72, Low activity). Some trainers/providers understood this and felt a media campaign normalising physical activity in older age would show they were valued, e.g., similar to the "This Girl Can" campaign [27]: *"If they can do that for girls, why can't they do it for older people"* (Jill, F, 40, Trainer).

3.2. Tackling Disadvantage

Older adults in low SES areas felt a strong sense of disadvantage, perceiving that those in higher SES areas received more acceptable and desirable physical activities:

They won't bring [Tai Chi] up here. They won't think of [people from local area] doing things like that! [. . .] they're the ones [in wealthier area] that'll get it. We wouldn't get it, you know [. . .] there's not one place doing Tai Chi [in local area], there's about three places [in wealthier area] doing it. (Linda, F, 68, Low activity)

Funding cuts in low SES areas had resulted in the loss of local facilities: *"We do miss our swimming pool"* (Sally, F, 78, Highly active); lack of services: *"There's nowhere round here to dance"* (Jo, F, 69, Low activity); and fear of loss of existing services: *"I'm trying to envisage what they, how they would access things and how they would go about it once [we] aren't there"* (Emma, F, 33, Provider).

Lack of individual resources seemed to impact attending physical activity sessions in low SES areas. Available transport was seen as unfit for purpose, with older adults feeling they needed to leave classes early to ensure they did not miss transport and consequently feeling vulnerable in unsafe neighbourhoods: *"[They] started coming when they wanted, so I was missing half the [class . . .] because I'd have to go outside and wait. And you don't want to be stood up there outside anything"* (Linda, F, 68, Low activity). Those with access to private transport did not have such issues with travelling to evening activities within low SES areas: *"Well not for where we would be going, because we'd only be going local, and I'd be driving[. . .] door to door, yeah"* (Diana, F, 71, Highly active).

Shared community resources were lost to other services, such as socialising spaces becoming offices: *"They used to go upstairs and have tea and biscuits [. . .] you know what it's like, funding"* (Jill, F, 40, Trainer). Trainers/providers found ways around their lack of resources with innovative use of existing services, e.g., ending a walk at a free coffee morning. However, the seeming inevitability of loss of services was also a focus within some delivery in an attempt to prepare older adults in low SES areas to cope when such loss occurred: *"Over the years, I've educated them. 'So, if I can't make it. If this building has to close [. . .] you know at home that you can do this'"* (James, M, 30, Trainer).

Replacing community venues with centralised facilities outside the area did not seem to be acceptable: *"Merge them and make something bigger, and then you can put more funding into that and make it more successful. But it just doesn't work"* (Emma, F, 33, Provider). Planners of such centralisation appeared unaware of the disadvantages that a lack of personal resources could have on older adults' ability to attend a centralised facility: *"To the leisure centre, their thing was 'Oh it's only down the road.' And it is only down the road, but not to maybe an older person who maybe doesn't travel, or has walked there, or isn't confident crossing main roads"* (Katie, F, 32, Provider).

3.3. Flexibility

Some providers mentioned that older adults seemed to lack flexibility around timetabling: *"If we have to change the instructor, or the time and the day, it kicks up such a fuss and we have to be very sympathetic to that"* (Katie, F, 32, Provider). Flexibility in older adults' thinking around changing plans or incorporating physical activity into their routine was in fact evident, particularly through first-hand experience: *"But now I see that I can be active"* (Al, M, 77, Highly active). However, flexibility could be disrupted when higher priority conflicts occurred, such as family commitments: *"I used to go walking, but it was a funny time. That was on a Thursday. My daughter comes on a Thursday"* (Julie, F, 72, Highly active). Some whose working life had consisted of hard physical jobs also seemed to struggle with now viewing physical activity as a leisure pursuit to be engaged in during their traditional leisure time of the weekend: *"I said, "Not Saturday! [when asked to go on a walk]"* (Kath, F, 77, Somewhat active).

3.4. Familiarity

Reframing unfamiliar movements with familiar terms improved acceptability of the physical activity itself:

> *They couldn't remember the names of the movements, so they made up their own names and they were things like, "pulling the beer pump" or "changing the baby's nappy," or "washing the car," but it made them, it helped them understand the [Tai Chi] movements, and as soon as that clicked in, that they renamed them, they could do the movements really comfortably.* (Phil, M, 46, Trainer)

Familiarity with trainers helped to build trust, and there was a keen sense of loss when familiar trainers left: *"It was really a smack in the teeth when she went"* (Linda, F, 68, Low activity). Social contact with familiar others seemed to be a primary driver for engaging in physical activity: *"Knowing people who go to it, that's the main thing"* (Sara, F, 74, Somewhat active). Fear of rejection in unfamiliar places adversely affected acceptability: *"If I sat there for an hour on my own and nobody came near me [. . .] I just couldn't cope with that. So that's why I don't go"* (Jo, F, 69, Low activity). However, some providers perceived a reluctance to travel beyond their familiar council area (ward) as something ingrained within the low SES community itself:

> *You find that they will go to something that's very, very near to them. But if you put the same class that they wanted on and you moved it to a different ward, they wouldn't want to travel. And that's not always easy to put something on in every ward. So, you will get that [. . .] where they just won't cross over [. . .] I don't know whether it's because they feel safe in their ward or if . . . they're being a traitor?* (Emma, F, 33, Provider)

3.5. Enjoyment

Providing and promoting opportunities for enjoyment was seen as key to acceptability:

> *Brand them as something else. Or put another spin on it, so people engage because it's social, it's fun, it's friends. The health, the physical activity and everything else is a by-product. That's something that might be our aim, but that's not how we sell it.* (Frank, M, 44, Trainer/Provider)

Life was not to be wasted on unenjoyable activities: *"You've got to enjoy what you're doing, or otherwise don't do it"* (Sally, F, 78, Highly active). When a regular physical activity was skipped, its absence was felt in both a lack of intrinsic enjoyment and also the lack of positive side effects usually experienced: *"You don't have the same energy I don't think [. . .] If I don't go [swimming], I do miss going"* (Shirley, F, 70, Active). Being immersed in physical activity helped some older adults to stay focused and enjoy living in the moment: *"It's fantastic . . . I'm living in the present moment"* (Al, M, 77, Highly active).

The anticipation of seeing friends and socializing within and around classes was integral: *"We enjoy one another's company while we're doing it, so that's the joyful part of it"* (Kevin, M, 71, Highly active); such social enjoyment could even help them to overlook physical ailments: *"You forget what's wrong with you when you've got a crowd of people"* (Grace, F, 94, Low activity). Anticipated enjoyment of an activity could also help some older adults to overcome environmental barriers in their low SES neighbourhood:

They were selling drugs down there [. . .] and [my friend] said, "I'm not going down there anymore." So, I started going, I got on my bike and went down on the bike on my own, yeah, and didn't mind cos I was enjoying it. (Mo, F, 89, Low activity)

For some older adults in low SES areas physical activity seemed to be a way to enjoy a simple freedom: *"It [cycling] feels like freedom to me, you know"* (Diana, F, 71, Highly active); something they felt they had not had much experience of in their working life and were now being afforded through physical activities: *"We were allowed to be ourselves. We were given permission to have fun"* (Olive, F, 70, Highly active).

3.6. Identity

How older adults in low SES areas identified with certain physical activities appeared to be important, e.g., one participant indicated that they disliked walking as an activity but were willing to join walks with a purpose (e.g., history, nature), as this participant noted about dancing: *"I've never been a dancer in my life [. . .] It's not me. I don't want to do it"*; but speaking on belly dancing: *"So I went, and it was a good laugh"* (Linda, F, 68, Low activity).

Identifying as physically active for some was related to hard physical jobs they no longer felt capable of: *"I think I'm past it"* (Susan, F, 80, Low activity). Some did not equate structured formal physical activity or exercise as something they would do in older age: *"Those days are over I think"* (Sam, M, 67, Active), preferring activities such as walking or gardening. For some, their sense of identity prevented involvement with activities provided by older-adult-based services: *"I don't FEEL like a pensioner [. . .] it's just not for me"* (Olive, F, 70, Highly active). Others still very much identified as active people, but on further investigation, they were referring to a sense of busyness in their schedule rather than being overly physically active: *"I don't think there's anything more that I could really do, if I think about it"* (Kath, F, 77, Somewhat active).

3.7. Group Cohesion

Being part of a cohesive group was important for maintaining physical activity: *"When you're with people that you know, you're more encouraged to go, aren't you? [. . .] because if you're on your own and you think, 'Oh I won't bother, I'll leave it'"* (Claire, F, 67, Somewhat active). Providers spoke of the process of a room full of strangers becoming a cohesive group:

That's a really lovely thing to see, when you start a new group, and you've got all these strangers around the room, and they kind of don't know each other, or some of them will know each other, and they don't know what they're doing, they don't know what's expected. And then over a period of time, you see it, something happens, a kind of, it settles, you know? It's like a cake in the oven, you know, isn't it? [laughing] You put all the ingredients together, and then magically it turns into a cake. (Fiona, F, 61, Trainer/Provider)

Group cohesion needed managing to incorporate new members: *"It does stop other people, if somebody doesn't make you welcome, you stop the class from growing"* (Sara, F, 74, Somewhat active).

3.8. Multi-Functionality

Attendance at physical activity sessions addressed multi-functional needs for older adults including social: *"Well, 50 per cent is activity, and 50 per cent is sociability with the people"* (Sara, F, 74, Somewhat active); or leisure interests: *"We [the walking group] go to the science museum and the other museums, you know, and I like that kind of thing [. . .] You're absorbing knowledge as well, you see, and I find that interesting"* (Liz, F, 74, Active). For others, solitary physical activity was acceptable only if it also addressed other needs: *"I'd walk up to the shops on my own alright but not to go out for a walk on my own"* (Mo, F, 89, Low activity). Multi-functionality sometimes hindered the intensity of physical activity, as noted by both trainers/providers and some more active older adults: *"We struggle to maintain a good walking pace when the people that walk with me are often interested in nature and stopping to* observe things" (Mary, F, 62, Trainer/Provider); "It drags me down when you're walking slow, waiting for people or walking in a group that's not walking, if you know what I mean [...] I want the walk" (Diana, F, 71, Highly active). However, maintenance was encouraged due to multi-functionality, e.g., walking to and from a sociable physical activity to meet social needs despite weather stopping much of the session activity, ensuring that the routine of attending was maintained and a couple of short walks still undertaken:

> If it was pouring down with rain we wouldn't say "Oh, we won't bother going to the club" you know, we'd still [walk] round. I mean if it's gardening, we wouldn't go out in the garden. We'd just sit there and have a cup of tea and a chat, you know, and then come home. (Ben, M, 74, Low activity)

Lack of multi-functionality coupled with limited resources could result in older adults in low SES areas pitting physical activity against other activities: " ... more to do with how that encroaches in my life balance of how much time I want to spend doing that, as against something else that I want to do" (Sam, M, 67, Active).

4. Discussion

This study explored individual perspectives on older adults' acceptability of physical activity provision from both older adults living in and trainers/providers working in low SES areas. The eight themes produced together show the varied and complex issues related to provision and engagement with physical activity for older adults in lower SES areas. The older adults often felt disadvantaged and undervalued when comparing themselves to older adults in higher SES areas and to younger people in general. Their sense of value increased when they felt that their needs were taken into consideration and when they were provided with physical activities deemed appealing to others.

Several studies have shown that reduced amenities and limited resources in low SES areas negatively impact engagement in leisure-time physical activity [6–8,28]. In the present study, trainers/providers working within low SES areas generally understood the negative impact limited resources had on older adults' ability to engage in physical activity and did their utmost to make the older adults who attended feel valued by listening and providing time for them all to talk, thereby providing social contact and promoting group cohesion. However, they often felt powerless in the face of the apparent lack of such understanding by facility management, who further compounded the disadvantages faced by older adults living in lower SES areas by centralising physical activity services, cancelling classes with little notice, and removing provision in low SES areas.

The feelings regarding inequality of provision in the current study are perhaps unsurprising, as it has been shown that parity of provision is often absent in low SES areas. A study of the spatial distribution of facilities [29] found low/medium SES areas contained fewer physical activity facilities overall and fewer free facilities than higher SES areas. A Spanish study [30] found such a lack of local convenient facilities negatively impacted the physical activity levels of older women (but not older men or younger adults) in lower SES areas. The lack of societal value older adults in lower SES areas experienced in the current study was stark when their classes were the first to be cancelled, when current provision was taken away, and when attractive provision was offered in more affluent neighbourhoods by the same provider but not in their neighbourhoods. Furthermore, the removal of vital social facilities within municipal buildings in low SES areas further illustrated the seeming lack of understanding of older adults' needs by facility management. To feel disregarded in such a manner was no inducement to engage in physical activity even though some trainers/providers tried to equip older adults with the knowledge to continue independently should local provision close. Trainers/providers also tried to tackle lack of social facilities as best they could with innovative use of existing free services, but such opportunities were rarely available. Furthermore, the removal of opportunities to socialise around physical activity sessions in the lower SES area facilities added further to the inequality by reducing the multi-functionality of the event, where older adults with limited resources may be forced to choose between attending a socially or physically beneficial activity.

The issue of these limited resources needs to be addressed in order to tackle such disadvantage. Lack of access to private or public transport, together with centralised services moved further afield, requires greater expenditure of both time and energy merely to attend a physical activity session, making engagement challenging for those with limited resources [26]. Furthermore, as noted in the current study, the impact of unreliable transport was compounded by feelings of vulnerability in unsafe neighbourhoods, again reducing the acceptability of attending physical activity sessions for many. It should be noted that, even though all participants lived in lower SES areas, actual level of income was not recorded in the current study. Given this, some participants may have had greater funds that increased their possible access to private transportation and other amenities further afield. The relationship between neighbourhood safety and leisure-time physical activity has been reported as a barrier to physical activity for older adults in low SES areas [9]. Some older adults in the current study suggested that the pleasure they derived from sessions was enough for them to overcome such environmental barriers but not for others they knew.

The perceived added value of group activities for lifestyle behaviour change has been noted as more important for low SES older adults than those of higher SES [28]. The current study suggests that facilitating strong social bonds and group cohesion helped older adults to maintain regular physical activity, perhaps due to a perceived obligation to group members [28]. Promotion of the social aspect of group physical activities may help older adults in low SES areas to identify more with the pleasure of leisure-time physical activity rather than to see it as hard work, something that many have had enough of. Although we did not collect data on how many physical activity classes or other social classes participants in the current study attended per week, such information may illustrate further the preferences for engaging socially or not within this target population. Social physical activity sessions did seem highly acceptable in low SES areas across the majority of participants regardless of their activity levels. This suggests that more sociable provision may encourage more older adults to leave their house, which is itself positively associated with higher levels of physical activity [7]. Focusing on social aspects rather than physical aspects of provision was also seen to be more acceptable to older adults in low SES areas by the trainers/providers who worked there, both in practice and in marketing. Such findings are in line with social goals being more relevant motivators to being physically active for older adults than younger adults [31].

4.1. Strengths and Limitations of Study

The multi-perspective aspect of this study gives insight into issues of acceptability of physical activity provision from both older adults and trainers/providers delivering physical activity in lower SES areas. This approach allowed us to see different facets of the same issue in an understudied context, which could inform future provision. The study was conducted in a city that is ranked third highest for deprivation in England [20] and recruited in areas with higher deprivation for older adults within that city. This use of an objective measure of SES for recruitment area took into account salient environmental and household issues specific to the study population, without experiencing possible underreporting of sensitive information, as can occur with individual measures of SES [32]. However, there was a broad range of education among older adult participants, with the majority having secondary school education or lower but two participants having PhDs. Collecting household income data may have illustrated differences in individual circumstances.

Older adults' activity levels used to describe the sample were defined in accordance with recommended guidelines; however, their self-report has limitations of lower accuracy compared to objective measures [33]. Although purposive sampling resulted in wide range of activity levels within older adults and a wide range of work sectors within trainers/providers, there was low gender and ethnic diversity. These latter two factors somewhat limit the insight gained, as does the focus on urban areas.

4.2. Implications

These findings suggest that providing multi-functional desirable physical activities that focus on fun, social, or leisure interests may allow older adults with limited resources to be physically active without sacrificing other desired activities. This approach may also capture more inactive older adults simply looking for fun, social activities who would not necessarily be drawn to a purely physical activity but who may nevertheless experience the health/wellbeing benefits as a by-product. Consistent, familiar, local provision may reduce expenditure of financial, physical, and mental resources whilst retaining social networks and encouraging maintenance of physical activity. Further research is required to confirm and quantify these findings in a larger, more diverse sample.

5. Conclusions

The present research sets out multiple facets of physical activity provision that are linked to acceptability of physical activity to older adults in low SES areas. To increase acceptability of physical activity for older adults in low SES areas, providers should address the lack of personal perceived value felt by many older adults. Equitable provision of physical activities addressing multiple needs (e.g., social, hobbies) may allow older adults with fewer resources to be physically active without sacrificing other needs. Such provision needs to be social, familiar, and enjoyable, so it may be perceived as a leisure-time activity. Facilitation of social interaction creates strong social bonds, potentially fostering maintenance of physical activities. Addressing these issues is likely to produce greater acceptability and thereby greater engagement in physical activity in this population.

Supplementary Materials: The following are available online at https://www.mdpi.com/article/10.3390/ijerph182211784/s1. Supplementary S1: Older Adults' Interview Schedule; Supplementary S2: Trainers/Providers' Interview Schedule

Author Contributions: Conceptualization, A.D.-F., D.P.F., and R.P.; methodology, A.D.-F., and R.P.; validation, A.D.-F., D.P.F., and R.P.; formal analysis, A.D.-F., R.P., and D.P.F.; data curation, A.D.-F., D.P.F.; writing—original draft preparation, A.D.-F.; writing—review and editing, A.D.-F., D.P.F., and R.P.; supervision, D.P.F. and R.P.; project administration, A.D.-F.; funding acquisition, A.D.-F. and D.P.F. All authors have read and agreed to the published version of the manuscript.

Funding: This research was funded by The University of Manchester President's Doctoral Scholarship Award granted to the first author.

Institutional Review Board Statement: The study was conducted according to the guidelines of the Declaration of Helsinki and approved by Ethics Committee 1 of the University of Manchester (Ref: 14391 15 January 2021).

Informed Consent Statement: Written informed consent was obtained from all subjects involved in the study.

Data Availability Statement: The data that support the findings of this study are available on reasonable request from the corresponding author. The data are not publicly available due to privacy or ethical restrictions.

Acknowledgments: We are grateful to all the participants for their time and openness as well as the local groups who facilitated engagement in our research: Age UK in Manchester, Age-Friendly Manchester, the Manchester Institute for Collaborative Research on Ageing (MICRA), and Manchester City Council who advertised the research project and/or allowed access to classes and groups to facilitate recruitment.

Conflicts of Interest: The authors declare no conflict of interest.

References

1. McPhee, J.S.; French, D.P.; Jackson, D.; Nazroo, J.; Pendleton, N.; Degens, H. Physical activity in older age: Perspectives for healthy ageing and frailty. *Biogerontology* **2016**, *17*, 567–580. [CrossRef] [PubMed]
2. UK Department of Health. *Start Active, Stay Active: A Report on Physical Activity for Health from the Four Home Countries' Chief Medical Officers*; UK Department of Health: London, UK, 2011. Available online: https://www.gov.uk/government/publications/start-active-stay-active-a-report-on-physical-activity-from-the-four-home-countries-chief-medical-officers (accessed on 20 September 2016).
3. Scholes, S.; Mindell, J. Physical activity in adults. In *Health for England 2012*; Craig, R., Mindell, J., Eds.; Health and Social Care Information Centre: Leeds, UK, 2013; Volume 1, Chapter 2; pp. 1–49. Available online: https://files.digital.nhs.uk/publicationimport/pub13xxx/pub13218/hse2012-ch2-phys-act-adults.pdf (accessed on 1 September 2016).
4. Scholes, S. *Health Survey for England 2016: Physical Activity in Adults*; Health and Social Care Information Centre: Leeds, UK, 2017. Available online: https://files.digital.nhs.uk/publication/m/3/hse16-adult-phy-act.pdf (accessed on 3 September 2020).
5. Public Health England. *Everybody Active, Every Day: An Evidence-Based Approach to Physical Activity*; Public Health England: London, UK, 2014. Available online: https://assets.publishing.service.gov.uk/government/uploads/system/uploads/attachment_data/file/374914/Framework_13.pdf (accessed on 20 September 2016).
6. Annear, M.J.; Cushman, G.; Gidlow, B. Leisure time physical activity differences among older adults from diverse socioeconomic neighborhoods. *Health Place* **2009**, *15*, 482–490. [CrossRef] [PubMed]
7. Fox, K.R.; Hillsdon, M.; Sharp, D.; Cooper, A.R.; Coulson, J.C.; Davis, M.; Harris, R.; McKenna, J.; Narici, M.; Stathi, A.; et al. Neighbourhood deprivation and physical activity in UK older adults. *Health Place* **2011**, *17*, 633–640. [CrossRef]
8. King, A.C. Interventions to promote physical activity by older adults. *J. Gerontol. A Biol. Sci. Med. Sci.* **2001**, *56*, 36–46. [CrossRef]
9. Gray, P.M.; Murphy, M.H.; Gallagher, A.M.; Simpson, E.E.A. Motives and barriers to physical activity among older adults of different socioeconomic status. *J. Aging Phys. Act.* **2015**, *24*, 419–429. [CrossRef] [PubMed]
10. McGowan, L.; Devereux-Fitzgerald, A.; Powell, R.; French, D.P. How acceptable do older adults find the concept of being physically active? A systematic review and meta-synthesis. *Int. Rev. Sport Exerc. Psychol.* **2018**, *11*, 1–24. [CrossRef]
11. Devereux-Fitzgerald, A.; Powell, R.; Dewhurst, A.; French, D.P. The acceptability of physical activity interventions to older adults: A systematic review and meta-synthesis. *Soc. Sci. Med.* **2016**, *158*, 14–23. [CrossRef]
12. Skivington, K.; Matthews, L.; Simpson, S.A.; Craig, P.; Baird, J.; Blazeby, J.M.; Boyd, K.A.; Craig, N.; French, D.P.; McIntosh, E.; et al. A new framework for developing and evaluating complex interventions: Update of Medical Research Council guidance. *Br. Med. J.* **2021**, *374*, n2061. [CrossRef]
13. Sekhon, M.; Cartwright, M.; Francis, J.J. Acceptability of healthcare interventions: A theoretical framework and proposed research agenda. *Br. J. Health Psychol.* **2018**, *23*, 519–531. [CrossRef]
14. Phoenix, C.; Orr, N. The multidimensionality of pleasure in later life. In *Physical Activity and Sport in Later Life: Critical Perspectives*; Tulle, E., Phoenix, C., Eds.; Palgrave Macmillan: London, UK, 2015.
15. Devereux-Fitzgerald, A.; McGowan, L.; Powell, R.; French, D.P. Making physical activity interventions acceptable to older people. In *The Palgrave Handbook of Ageing and Physical Activity Promotion*; Nyman, S.R., Ed.; Palgrave Macmillan: Cham, Switzerland, 2018; pp. 291–311. [CrossRef]
16. Franco, M.R.; Tong, A.; Howard, K.; Sherrington, C.; Ferreira, P.H.; Pinto, R.Z.; Ferreira, M.L. Older people's perspectives on participation in physical activity: A systematic review and thematic synthesis of qualitative literature. *Br. J. Sports Med.* **2015**, *49*, 1221–1222. [CrossRef]
17. Fox, K.R.; Stathi, A.; McKenna, J.; Davis, M.G. Physical activity and mental well-being in older people participating in the Better Ageing Project. *Eur. J. App. Physiol.* **2007**, *100*, 591–602. [CrossRef]
18. Hawley-Hague, H.; Horne, M.; Campbell, M.; Demack, S.; Skelton, D.; Todd, C. Multiple levels of influence on older adults' attendance and adherence to community exercise classes. *Gerontologist* **2013**, *54*, 599–610. [CrossRef]
19. Kendall, M.; Murray, S.A.; Carduff, E.; Worth, A.; Harris, F.; Lloyd, A.; Cavers, D.; Grant, L.; Boyd, K.; Sheikh, A. Use of multiperspective qualitative interviews to understand patients' and carers' beliefs, experiences, and needs. *Br. Med. J.* **2009**, *339*, b4122. [CrossRef]
20. Department for Communities and Local Government. *English Indices of Deprivation 2010*; Department for Communities and Local Government: London, UK, 2011. Available online: https://www.gov.uk/government/statistics/english-indices-of-deprivation-2010 (accessed on 20 October 2014).
21. Hildebrand, M.; Neufeld, P. Recruiting older adults into a physical activity promotion program: Active Living Every Day offered in a naturally occurring retirement community. *Gerontologist* **2009**, *49*, 702–710. [CrossRef]
22. Braun, V.; Clarke, V. Using thematic analysis in psychology. *Qual. Res. Psychol.* **2006**, *3*, 77–101. [CrossRef]
23. Ritchie, J.; Spencer, L. Qualitative data analysis for applied policy research. In *Analyzing Qualitative Data*; Bryman, A., Burgess, R.G., Eds.; Routledge: London, UK, 1994; pp. 173–194.
24. Ormston, R.; Spencer, L.; Barnard, M.; Snape, D. The foundations of qualitative research. In *Qualitative Research Practice: A Guide for Social Science Students & Researchers*, 2nd ed.; Edited by Ritchie, J., Lewis, J., Nicholls, C.M., Ormston, R., Eds.; Sage: London, UK, 2014.
25. Spencer, L.; Ritchie, J.; O'Connor, W.; Morrell, G.; Ormston, R. Analysis in practice. In *Qualitative Research Practice: A Guide for Social Science Students and Researchers*; Ritchie, J., Lewis, J., Nicholls, C.M., Ormston, R., Eds.; Sage: London, UK, 2013; pp. 295–345.

26. Devereux-Fitzgerald, A.; Powell, R.; French, D.P. Conflating time and energy: Views from older adults in lower socioeconomic status areas on physical activity. *J. Aging Phys. Act.* **2017**, *26*, 506–513. [CrossRef]
27. Sport England. *This Girl Can*; Sport England: London, UK, 2015. Available online: https://www.sportengland.org/campaigns-and-our-work/this-girl-can (accessed on 1 September 2016).
28. Bukman, A.J.; Teuscher, D.; Feskens, E.J.M.; van Baak, M.A.; Meershoek, A.; Renes, R.J. Perceptions on healthy eating, physical activity and lifestyle advice: Opportunities for adapting lifestyle interventions to individuals with low socioeconomic status. *BMC Public Health* **2014**, *14*, 1036. [CrossRef]
29. Estabrooks, P.A.; Lee, R.E.; Gyurscik, N.C. Resources for physical activity participation: Does availability and accessibility differ by neighborhood Socioeconomic Status? *Ann. Behav. Med.* **2003**, *25*, 100–104. [CrossRef]
30. Pascual, C.; Regidor, E.; Alvarez-del Arco, D.; Alejos, B.; Santos., J.M.; Calle, M.E.; Martinez, D. Sports facilities in Madrid explain the relationship between neighbourhood economic context and physical inactivity in older people, but not in younger adults: A case study. *J. Epidemiol. Community Health* **2013**, *67*, 788–794. [CrossRef]
31. Steltenpohl, C.N.; Shuster, M.; Peist, E.; Pham, A.; Mikels, J.A. Me time, or we time? Age differences in motivation for exercise. *Gerontologist* **2018**, *59*, 709–717. [CrossRef]
32. Gidlow, C.; Halley Johnston, L.; Crone, D.; Ellisa, N.; James, D. A systematic review of the relationship between socio-economic position and physical activity. *Health Educ. J.* **2006**, *65*, 338–367. [CrossRef]
33. Sallis, J.F.; Saelens, B.E. Assessment of physical activity by self-report: Status, limitations and future directions. *Res. Q. Exerc. Sport* **2000**, *71*, 1–14. [CrossRef] [PubMed]

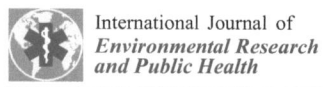

Article

Healthcare Professionals Promotion of Physical Activity with Older Adults: A Survey of Knowledge and Routine Practice

Conor Cunningham [1,*] and Roger O'Sullivan [1,2]

1. Institute of Public Health, Belfast BT1 4JH, UK
2. Bamford Centre for Mental Health and Wellbeing, Ulster University, Belfast BT37 0QB, UK
* Correspondence: conor.cunningham@publichealth.ie

Abstract: Healthcare professionals have a key role in promoting physical activity, particularly among populations at greatest risk of poor health due to physical inactivity. This research aimed to develop our understanding of healthcare professionals knowledge, decision making and routine practice of physical activity promotion with older adults. A cross-sectional survey was conducted with practicing healthcare professionals in general practice, physiotherapy, occupational therapy and nursing in Ireland and Northern Ireland. We received 347 eligible responses, with 70.3% of all respondents agreeing that discussing physical activity is their job and 30.0% agreeing that they have received suitable training to initiate conversations with patients about physical activity. Awareness of the content and objectives of national guidelines for physical activity varied considerably across the health professions surveyed. Less than a third of respondents had a clear plan on how to initiate discussions about physical activity in routine practice with older adults. Assessment of physical activity was not routine, neither was signposting to physical activity supports. Considering the COVID-19 pandemic and its implications, 81.6% of all respondents agreed that healthcare professionals can play an increased role in promoting physical activity to older adults as part of routine practice. Appropriate education, training and access to resources are essential for supporting healthcare professionals promotion of physical activity in routine practice. Effective physical activity promotion in healthcare settings has the potential for health benefits at a population level, particularly in older adult populations.

Keywords: physical activity; healthcare professionals; older adults; theoretical domains framework; policy; behaviour change

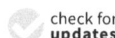

Citation: Cunningham, C.; O'Sullivan, R. Healthcare Professionals Promotion of Physical Activity with Older Adults: A Survey of Knowledge and Routine Practice. *Int. J. Environ. Res. Public Health* **2021**, *18*, 6064. https://doi.org/10.3390/ijerph18116064

Academic Editor: Paul B. Tchounwou

Received: 16 April 2021
Accepted: 29 May 2021
Published: 4 June 2021

Publisher's Note: MDPI stays neutral with regard to jurisdictional claims in published maps and institutional affiliations.

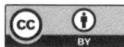

Copyright: © 2021 by the authors. Licensee MDPI, Basel, Switzerland. This article is an open access article distributed under the terms and conditions of the Creative Commons Attribution (CC BY) license (https://creativecommons.org/licenses/by/4.0/).

1. Introduction

The health benefits of physical activity for older adults are well established [1]. There is strong evidence that physical activity contributes to increased physical function, reduced impairment, independent living, and improved quality of life in both healthy and frail older adults [2]. International guidelines recommend that all older adults (65+ years) should aim to do at least 150–300 min of moderate intensity or 75–150 min of vigorous intensity aerobic activity throughout the week, with muscle strengthening and multicomponent balance training on 2 or more days per week [3]. In addition to recommending that all older adults should undertake regular physical activity, these guidelines also emphasize the benefits to older adults of 'moving more' and sitting less throughout the day, as doing some physical activity is better than none [3]. However, for many older adults, ageing is defined by rapid declines in levels of physical activity, loss of mobility and functional independence, and premature morbidity [4]. Therefore, this stage of life represents an important period for promoting physical activity to improve functions of daily living and slow progression of disease and disability [5].

Effective national action to reverse trends in inactivity across the life course requires a 'systems-based' approach, with action across different sectors [6]. As part of this approach, healthcare services can play an important role by implementing systems for patient assessment and counselling, and by strengthening the provision of and access to opportunities and programmes that enable older adults to increase their levels of physical activity [7]. Healthcare professionals play a central role in the promotion of a variety of health behaviours and are ideally positioned to promote physical activity [8]. Evidence suggests that they can positively impact patient behaviour by routinely assessing physical activity levels and by using brief practical interventions (advice or counselling on how to initiate and maintain healthy behaviours) with links to community-based support for behaviour change [9]. These are key actions in promoting health enhancing physical activity to reduce the incidence of chronic disease and/or to manage a range of chronic conditions and weight maintenance [10]. Indeed, recent healthcare policy developments on the island of Ireland (Ireland and Northern Ireland) recognize that preventing and reducing chronic disease across the life course by addressing inactivity (amongst other modifiable risk factors) requires a cultural shift on improving health and wellbeing through strategies that focus on health promotion and disease prevention [11].

Enhancing our understanding of current practice in relation to physical activity promotion in the health services is crucial to inform the development of evidence-based strategies for improving uptake of policy into practice. Previous research suggests that healthcare professionals instigate brief physical activity interventions opportunistically in a quarter of appropriate instances [9] and there is a disparity between the development of guidelines for physical activity and their dissemination and integration into routine clinical practice for many healthcare professionals [12–14]. Barriers to physical activity promotion have been reported by healthcare professionals, including lack of awareness, expertise, and lack of time and incentive [8]. It is unclear what level of knowledge around physical activity exists across a broad range of healthcare professionals on the island of Ireland, and to what extent physical activity promotion with older adults is involved in decision making in routine practice. This research is therefore focused on developing our understanding of healthcare professionals approaches to promoting physical activity to older adults in Ireland and Northern Ireland by evaluating their knowledge of current physical activity guidelines and exploring the factors which may influence their clinical judgements and decision making in promoting physical activity to older adults in routine practice. As this research took place during the COVID-19 pandemic, healthcare professionals perceptions of the implications of the public health and social measures for older adults' levels of physical activity, and their resultant behaviour(s) related to physical activity promotion with older adults in routine practice were also explored.

2. Materials and Methods

2.1. Sample and Eligibility

This was a cross-sectional study of practicing healthcare professionals in general practice, physiotherapy, occupational therapy and nursing in Ireland and Northern Ireland in 2020. Healthcare professionals who were not registered to practice in one of these four professional groups, those who were retired, working outside of Ireland or Northern Ireland, or who did not have clinical contact with older adults (defined as ≥65 years) as part of routine care were excluded from the study.

2.2. Survey Tool

A 43-item (3-section) survey was developed using the theoretical domains framework (TDF). The TDF is an integrative framework of theories of behaviour change developed to identify influences on healthcare professional behaviour in the implementation of evidence-based recommendations [15]. It has been used extensively to identify barriers and facilitators for individual uptake of evidence-based practices and for implementation design and research [16].

Section 1 of the survey captured demographic and employment data as well as healthcare professionals self-reported levels of physical activity, knowledge of physical activity guidelines and awareness of resources to facilitate knowledge and practice development. Section 2 assessed TDF domains of healthcare professional's behaviour in assessment, discussion, and prescription of physical activity in routine practice. Healthcare professionals perceptions of the implications of the COVID-19 pandemic on older adults' levels of physical activity and views on the role of physical activity promotion to older adults in light of the pandemic were also examined. Section 3 of the survey used clinical vignettes (3 for each healthcare profession) to enable healthcare professionals to self-report routine practice in relation to physical activity promotion with older adults. Analysis and findings for Section 3 of the survey are reported in a separate publication.

2.3. Survey Piloting and Procedure

A research project advisory group ($N = 10$) participated in pilot testing, refinement, and approval of the survey. This group included appointed representatives of the Royal College of General Practitioners in Northern Ireland and the Irish College of General Practitioners in Ireland; the Chartered Society of Physiotherapy in Northern Ireland and the Irish Society of Chartered Physiotherapists in Ireland; the Royal College of Nursing in Northern Ireland and the Department of Public Health Nursing in Ireland; and the Royal College of Occupational Therapists in Northern Ireland and the Association of Occupational Therapists Ireland. The survey was live for a 2-month period from mid-August to mid-October 2020, during which time the link to the survey was promoted through focused email distribution and promoted widely on social media.

2.4. Data Analysis

All eligible returned surveys were included in the analysis regardless of missing data; consequently, the number of total responses for each survey item is varied. Descriptive and explorative analysis of the data were performed using IBM SPSS V.24 (IBM Inc., Armonk, NY, USA). Descriptive statistics were used to describe data from the survey reporting frequencies of responses. Pearson's chi squared tests were used to compare knowledge of guidelines for physical activity with assessment, discussion, prescription, and signposting of physical activity in routine practice. Knowledge of the guidelines was classified by dividing the participants into two groups: (1) those who correctly recalled three specific components of the physical activity guidelines for older adults (number of minutes per week of moderate intensity physical activity, vigorous intensity physical activity, and the number of days of strength, balance, and flexibility activities recommended for optimal health benefits); and (2) those who indicated that they did not know the guidelines, or who incorrectly recalled one or more specific component of physical activity guidelines for older adults. Statistical significance was set at p value <0.05.

3. Results

3.1. Participant Characteristics

In total, 573 responses were received. Of these, 143 did not meet the inclusion criteria, and a further 83 did not complete components of the survey required to be included in subsequent analysis. A total of 347 respondents met the inclusion criteria and their responses were included in subsequent analysis. Participant characteristics are presented in Table 1. Of the respondents, 44 (12.7%) were male and 299 (86.2%) were female. Three quarters of respondents (74.4%) were healthcare professionals practicing in Ireland. Nearly half of all respondents (49.0%) were physiotherapists. The proportion of all respondents who reported that they had 26+ years of practice experience was 27.4% ($n = 95$). Most respondents worked in the public sector (80.7%, $n = 280$). The proportion of respondents who achieved the recommended level of moderate intensity physical activity over a week was 40.6% ($n = 141$).

Table 1. Characteristics of survey participants.

	All Respondents		General Practice		Physiotherapy		Occupational Therapy		Nursing	
	N	%	N	%	N	%	N	%	N	%
Professional Affiliation										
General practitioner	36	10.4								
Physio-therapist	170	49.0								
Occupational therapist	103	29.7								
Nurse	38	11.0								
Gender										
Male	44	12.7	14	38.9	22	12.9	8	7.8		
Female	299	86.2	20	55.6	147	86.5	95	92.2	37	97.4
Prefer not to say	4	1.2	2	5.6	1	0.6			1	2.6
Years qualified										
0–5	39	11.2			18	10.6	21	20.4		
6–10	52	15.0	4	11.1	24	14.1	22	21.4	2	5.3
11–15	59	17.0	5	13.9	31	18.2	19	18.4	4	10.5
16–20	49	14.1	6	16.7	30	17.6	10	9.7	3	7.9
21–25	53	15.3	7	19.4	32	18.8	8	7.8	6	15.8
26+	95	27.4	14	38.9	35	20.6	23	22.3	23	60.5
Healthcare setting										
Primary	128	36.9	27	75	61	35.9	32	31.1	8	21.1
Secondary	62	17.9	7	19.4	32	18.8	17	16.5	6	15.8
Other	157	45.2	2	5.6	77	45.3	54	52.4	24	63.2
Health sector										
Public	280	80.7	33	91.7	141	82.9	83	80.6	23	60.5
Private	46	13.3	3	8.4	23	13.5	13	12.6	7	18.4
Other	21	6.1			6	3.5	7	6.8	8	21.1
Region										
Northern Ireland	89	25.6	14	38.9	59	34.7	10	9.7	6	15.8
Ireland	258	74.4	22	61.1	111	65.3	93	90.3	32	84.2
Total	347	100.0	36	100.0	170	100.0	103	100.0	38	100.0
Physical activity levels *										
Active	141	40.6	18	50.0	76	44.7	32	31.1	15	39.5
Inactive	205	59.1	17	47.2	94	55.3	71	68.9	23	60.5
Total	346	99.7	35	97.2	170	100	103	100	38	100

* Measured by Single Item Metric [17].

3.2. Knowledge, Understanding and Use of Physical Activity Guidelines

Responders were asked how aware they were of the content and objectives of national guidelines in their jurisdiction. Of all respondents, 42.7% ($n = 148$) (62.9% of physiotherapists, 34.2% of nurses, 22.2% of general practitioners and 19.4% of occupational therapists) agreed that they were aware of the content and objectives of national guidelines for physical activity in their jurisdiction (Table 2). Of all respondents, 35.4% ($n = 123$) agreed that they were aware of the content and objectives of national guidelines for physical activity for older adults in their jurisdiction. The percentage of those that 'agreed' varied considerably across the healthcare professions surveyed (Table 2).

Table 2. Participant's awareness of physical activity guidelines and resources.

Survey Question *	Answer	All Respondents		General Practice		Physiotherapy		Occupational Therapy		Nursing	
		N	%	N	%	N	%	N	%	N	%
I am aware of the content and objectives of national guidelines for physical activity in my jurisdiction	Agree	148	42.7	8	22.2	107	62.9	20	19.4	13	34.2
	Somewhat agree	111	32.0	12	33.3	35	20.6	44	42.7	20	52.6
	Neither agree nor disagree	13	3.7	3	8.3	3	1.8	5	4.9	2	5.3
	Somewhat disagree	19	5.5	1	2.8	4	2.4	13	12.6	1	2.6
	Disagree	20	5.8	6	16.7	2	1.2	12	11.7		
	Not stated	36	10.4	6	16.7	19	11.2	9	8.7	2	5.3
I am aware of the content and objectives of national guidelines for physical activity for older adults in my jurisdiction	Agree	123	35.4	8	22.2	89	52.4	17	16.5	9	23.7
	Somewhat agree	124	35.7	7	19.4	52	30.6	43	41.7	22	57.9
	Neither agree nor disagree	17	4.9	4	11.1	3	1.8	7	6.8	3	7.9
	Somewhat disagree	24	6.9	4	11.1	5	2.9	14	13.6	1	2.6
	Disagree	23	6.6	7	19.4	2	1.2	13	12.6	1	2.6
	Not stated	36	10.4	6	16.7	19	11.2	9	8.7	2	5.3
Awareness of specific component(s) of physical activity guidelines for older adults											
Do you know how many minutes of moderate intensity physical activity that the national guidelines recommend per week for older adults in your jurisdiction? Correct answer: 150	Yes	212	61.1	15	41.7	134	78.8	44	42.7	19	50.0
	Correctly answered **	170	49.0	9	25.0	120	70.6	30	29.1	11	28.9
	No	94	27.1	15	41.7	15	8.8	49	47.6	15	39.5
	Not stated	41	11.8	6	16.7	21	12.4	10	9.7	4	10.5
Do you know how many minutes of vigorous intensity physical activity that the national guidelines per week for older adults in your jurisdiction? Correct answer: 75	Yes	134	38.6	7	19.4	94	55.3	20	19.4	13	34.2
	Correctly answered **	95	27.4	2	5.6	76	44.7	12	11.7	5	13.2
	No	171	49.3	23	63.9	55	32.4	71	68.9	22	57.9
	Not stated	42	12.1	6	16.7	21	12.4	12	11.7	3	7.9

Table 2. Cont.

Survey Question *	Answer	All Respondents		General Practice		Physiotherapy		Occupational Therapy		Nursing	
		N	%	N	%	N	%	N	%	N	%
Do you know how many days per week that national guidelines in your jurisdiction recommend older adults perform strength, balance, and flexibility training	Yes	188	54.2	10	27.8	123	72.4	32	31.1	23	60.5
	Correctly answered **	179	51.6	9	25.0	117	68.8	28	27.2	22	57.9
	No	121	34.9	20	55.6	28	16.5	61	59.2	12	31.6
	Not stated	38	11.0	6	16.7	19	11.2	10	9.7	3	7.9
Correctly answered all 3 questions **		85	24.5	2	5.6	68	40.0	11	10.7	4	10.5
Awareness of resources											
I am aware of resources (i.e., online resources and toolkits) to facilitate my knowledge development and practice of discussions/ assessment / prescription of physical activity with patients as a part of routine care	Yes	165	47.6	4	11.1	109	64.1	34	33.0	18	47.4
	No	141	40.6	26	72.2	40	23.5	60	58.3	15	39.5
	Not stated	41	11.8	6	16.7	21	12.4	9	8.7	5	13.2

* Questions linked to 'Knowledge' domain of TDF ** Of those who replied 'Yes' and correctly recalled how many minutes/days when prompted.

Responders were also asked about their knowledge of three specific components of physical activity recommendations for older adults (number of minutes per week of moderate intensity physical activity, vigorous intensity physical activity, and the number of days of strength, balance, and flexibility activities recommended for optimal health benefits). Of all respondents, 61.1% ($n = 212$) reported that they knew how many weekly minutes of moderate intensity physical activity were recommended for older adults, and 38.6% ($n = 134$) of all respondents reported that they knew how many minutes of weekly vigorous intensity physical activity were recommended for older adults. However, when prompted, 49% ($n = 170$) correctly recalled the number of minutes of moderate intensity activity, and 27.4% ($n = 95$) correctly recalled the number of minutes of vigorous activity. 54.2% ($n = 188$) of all respondents reported that they knew how many days per week older adults were recommended to perform strength, balance, and flexibility training. The proportion who correctly recalled the number of days when prompted was 51.6% ($n = 179$). Of all respondents, 24.5% ($n = 85$) correctly recalled all three specific components of physical activity guidelines for older adults (Table 2).

Most respondents (64.6%) agreed that physical activity guidelines have a place in routine practice. However, only 26.5% of physiotherapists, 15.8% of nurses, 14.0% of occupational therapists, and 5.6% of general practitioners agreed that there is sufficient time allocated to implement physical activity guidelines for adults/older adults in day-to-day work (Table S1).

3.3. Awareness of Resources

Of all respondents, 47.6% ($n = 165$) (64.1% of physiotherapists, 47.4% of nurses, 33.0% of occupational therapists and 11.1% of general practitioners) reported that they were aware of resources to facilitate their knowledge development and practice of assessment/discussion/prescription of physical activity with patients as a part of routine care. The most frequently cited resources included government health department websites, professional body websites and health profession specific websites, and training programmes and research projects with online physical activity resources and toolkits (Figure 1).

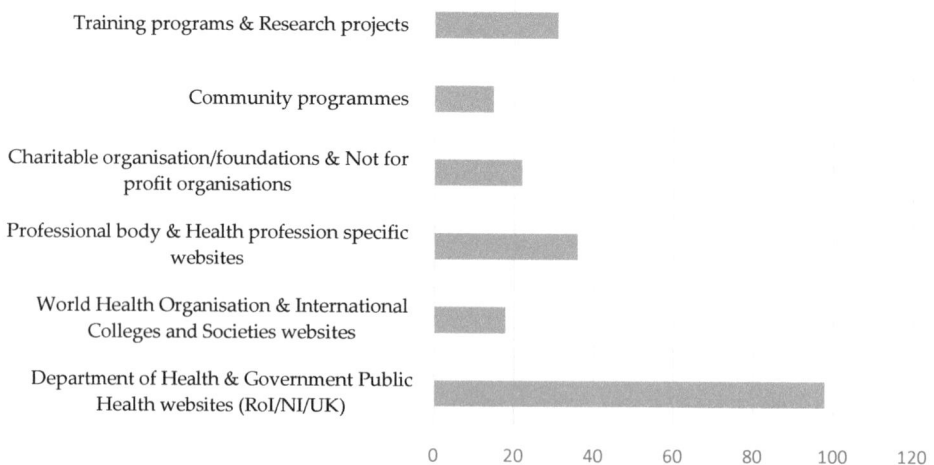

Figure 1. Resources accessed by participants for knowledge development of physical activity promotion.

3.4. Theoretical Domains of Health Professionals Behaviour

Table S1 shows the theoretical domains of healthcare professional's behaviour in assessment, discussion, and prescription of physical activity in routine practice.

3.4.1. Assessment of Patient's Physical Activity Levels

Responders were asked about their use of screening tools to measure patients' physical activity levels. Nearly half of all respondents (48.7%, $n = 169$) reported that they 'never' formally assess whether a patient is active or inactive as part of routine practice. The proportion who reported that they 'sometimes', 'usually', or 'always' assess whether a patient is active or inactive was 40.0% ($n = 139$). A variety a functional assessment tools (e.g., the Timed Up and Go (TUG) test, 6-min walk test), questionnaire based (e.g., General Practice Physical Activity Questionnaire (GPPAQ)) and device-based measures of physical activity (e.g., pedometers) were reported. Having knowledge of three specific components of physical activity guidelines for older adults was significantly associated with formally assessing whether a patient is active or inactive as part of routine practice (Table S1).

3.4.2. Discussing Physical Activity with Patients

Responders were asked if they considered it a part of their professional role to promote physical activity to patients. Most respondents (70.3%, $n = 244$) agreed that discussing physical activity with patients was part of their work as a healthcare professional. Many (74.1%, $n = 257$) 'agreed', or 'somewhat agreed' that it was easy to remember to discuss physical activity with patients (74.1%, $n = 257$) and that they were confident that they could discuss physical activity as part of routine practice even when the patient was not motivated (72%, $n = 250$) or when there was little time (63.8%, $n = 221$). Overall, 30.0% of all respondents ($n = 104$) agreed that they had received suitable training to initiate conversations with patients about physical activity. This percentage was higher for physiotherapists (44.1%) (Table S1). We found that 36.1% of general practitioners, 21.4% of occupational therapists, and 23.7% of nurses did not agree that they have received suitable training to initiate conversations with patients about physical activity.

3.4.3. Discussing Physical Activity with Older Adults

Most respondents (68.0%, $n = 236$) agreed that discussing physical activity with older adults was part of their work as a health professional, with the majority 'agreeing', or 'somewhat agreeing' that it is something they do automatically (67.6%, $n = 233$) and is useful (82.4%, $n = 286$). Many 'agreed', or 'somewhat agreed' that they were aware of how to initiate conversations about physical activity with older adults (83.5%, $n = 290$), that they had the skills to initiate conversations with older adults about physical activity (80.1%, $n = 278$) and that it was something that they typically did within their organization (72.1%, $n = 250$). There was a significant association between having knowledge of three specific components of physical activity guidelines for older adults and initiating conversations with patients about physical activity as part of routine practice (Table S1). However, even though many respondents agreed that that they intended to discuss physical activity in their next consultation/appointment with an older adult as part of routine care (55.0%, $n = 191$), fewer agreed that they had a clear plan on how to initiate discussions about physical activity in routine practice with older adults (30.5%, $n = 106$).

3.4.4. Physical Activity Prescription and Signposting

Responders were asked how often they refer/signpost patients through referral programmes or community-based schemes. We found that 12.1% of respondents 'always' signposted patients to other physical activity services (i.e., exercise referral programmes/community-based physical activity initiatives). Having knowledge of three specific components of physical activity guidelines for older adults was significantly associated with signposting patients to other physical activity services as part of routine practice (Table S1). Most physiotherapists (64.1%), occupational therapists (63.1%), general practitioners (61.2%), and 50.0% of nurses reported that they 'sometimes' or 'usually' signposted patients to other physical activity services. The physical activity services that they 'sometimes', 'usually', or 'always' signposted to patients included exercise referral programmes; community-based active retirement groups; community-based healthcare professional follow-up (e.g., fall prevention groups, community physiotherapy/occupational therapy services); online self-management groups/virtual classes and resources. Most respondents (68.6%) agreed that assessing/discussing/prescribing physical activity with an older adult as part of routine practice would benefit the public health agenda. 23.3% of occupational therapists, 21.1% of nurses and 2.8% of general practitioners agreed that they were supported to use physical activity assessment/discussions/prescription in everyday practice. This number was higher for physiotherapists (38.8%).

3.5. Older Adults' Physical Activity and the COVID-19 Pandemic

To explore healthcare professionals understanding of the potential impact of public health restrictions on older adults' levels of physical activity, and their resultant behaviour(s) related to physical activity promotion with older adults in routine practice, the following questions were asked (see Table 3). The proportion of all respondents who indicated that the public health and social measures introduced to prevent the spread of COVID-19 had reduced older adults' levels of physical activity was 71.2%, and considering this, 81.6% of all respondents agreed that healthcare professionals can play an increased role in promoting physical activity to older adults. Overall, 84.7% stated that they were 'more likely' (47.8%), or the 'same as usual' (36.9%) to discuss physical activity with older adults as part of routine practice considering the COVID-19 pandemic and its implications.

Table 3. The COVID-19 pandemic: implications for older adults' physical activity.

Survey Question	Answer	All Respondents		General Practice		Physiotherapy		Occupational Therapy		Nursing	
		N	%	N	%	N	%	N	%	N	%
Public health and social measures introduced to prevent the spread of COVID-19 have reduced older adults' levels of physical activity	Agree	247	71.2	20	55.6	123	72.4	79	76.7	25	65.8
	Somewhat agree	52	15.0	5	13.9	27	15.9	11	10.7	9	23.7
	Neither agree nor disagree	6	1.7	2	5.6	1	0.6	2	1.9	1	2.6
	Somewhat disagree	6	1.7	3	3.8			2	1.9	1	2.6
	Disagree										
	Not stated	36	10.4	6	16.7	19	11.2	9	8.7	2	5.3
In light of the COVID-19 pandemic—do you think that health professionals can play an increased role in promoting physical activity to older adults?	Yes	283	81.6	24	66.7	145	85.3	87	84.5	27	71.1
	No	5	1.4	2	5.6	6	3.5	1	1.0	2	5.3
	Don't know	21	6.1	3	8.3			6	5.8	6	15.8
	Not stated	38	11.0	7	19.4	19	11.2	9	8.7	3	7.9
Considering the COVID-19 pandemic—how likely are you to discuss physical activity with older adults as part of routine practice?	More likely	166	47.8	12	33.3	79	46.5	56	54.4	19	50.0
	Same as usual	128	36.9	15	41.7	64	37.6	35	34.0	14	36.8
	Less likely	16	4.6	3	8.3	7	4.1	3	2.9	3	7.9
	Not stated	37	10.7	6	16.7	20	11.8	9	8.7	2	5.3

4. Discussion

Healthcare professionals play a pivotal role in educating patients about the benefits of being more active and motivating their patients to engage in a more active lifestyle [18,19]. In this study most respondents agreed that discussing physical activity is their job (TDF domain: Social/Professional Role and Identity), and that it is easy to remember to do (TDF domain: Memory, Attention & Decision processes). However, the majority had not received suitable training in initiating discussions about physical activity with patients (TDF domain: Skills). Our survey also shows that many healthcare professionals are unaware of current guidelines for physical activity in older adults (TDF domain: Knowledge)—one in four correctly answered questions about the content of these guidelines, and less than a third of respondents had a clear plan on how to initiate discussions about physical activity in routine practice with older adults (TDF domain: Behavioural Regulation).

The results of this survey have identified a range of theoretical domains that can be targeted to support healthcare professionals in their role of promoting active lifestyle change with patients. In particular, the domains of Knowledge, Skills and Behavioural Regulation were identified. These domains map directly onto the 'Capability' component of the COM-B model of behaviour change [20]. Building healthcare professionals' 'Capability' to promote physical activity in routine practice through 'Knowledge' development: appropriate education on guidelines for physical activity in prevention and treatment of disease is essential. In this study, having a detailed knowledge and recall of physical activity guidelines for older adults was associated with formal assessment, initiating discussion, and referral/signposting to physical activity services as part of routine practice. Building capability through 'Skill' development: relevant training on initiating discussions/brief interventions to support patients with behavioural change (perhaps through motivational interviewing) is equally important. Evidence suggests that brief practical interventions by clinicians may improve short and long-term engagement with active lifestyles [21] and that components of motivational interviewing are central to this approach as a theory consistent and evidence-based technique to strengthen an individual's motivation for change [22].

The recently introduced Making Every Contact Count (MECC) strategy places the responsibility for providing brief (and opportunistic) interventions on all healthcare professionals who may have patient contact in Ireland and Northern Ireland. By integrating MECC at the initial/undergraduate level it is planned that brief interventions will become central to many consultations [23]. In this survey most respondents were fully qualified with regular patient contact for more than 6 years, which suggests that continuing education/professional development on physical activity promotion will be crucial to maximise their impact on and support for sustained behaviour change with their patients. This finding is consistent with other studies that have highlighted the need for postgraduate training for healthcare professionals to address health behaviour change [23,24], but also the need to integrate physical activity training and its relationship with health at an undergraduate level. Several reports indicate that this issue is now receiving greater attention in undergraduate curricula [25,26].

Many healthcare professionals surveyed never formally assess whether a patient is active or inactive as a part of routine practice. In part, this may reflect the level of training and support that healthcare professionals surveyed have received on physical activity promotion broadly, and on physical assessment more specifically. The routine assessment of physical activity (and sedentary behaviour) in the health system is the basis for the surveillance of physical inactivity as a risk factor [27]. Assessing a patient's level of physical activity can provide a valuable insight into health status and is an essential first step that can lead to important intervention opportunities, if appropriate. Those who reported that they assess physical activity and/or functional status in older adults used a variety of tools and resources. Whereas the use of tools to support the systematic screening and delivery of brief interventions is recommended, some have advocated the use of a standardised physical activity tool as a 'vital sign' in patients' consultations, that should be a standard of care for all patient visits with the potential to highlight inactivity and prompt a brief intervention (counselling or referral) [28].

Few respondents 'always' signposted patients to other physical activity services (i.e., exercise referral programmes/community-based physical activity initiatives). The majority reported that they did this 'usually' or 'sometimes'. Raising awareness of community resources (passive or active signposting) or prescribing activity as a means of referral is seen as a 'formal' acknowledgement of the problem (inactivity) and provides both a legitimacy to the issue and an opportunity to do something about it. Previous research has suggested that patients 'like' the option of being connected to resources on specific physical activity opportunities by a health professional, to consider and potentially follow up on [29].

How the topic is raised and linked to a patient's specific health conditions is central to patient acceptance to the topic [29], highlighting again the need for specific and ongoing education and training on initiating discussions and delivering brief interventions as part of routine care. Research suggests that the 'motivation' provided by a healthcare professional is key to whether a patient accepts offers of being signposted to community physical activity opportunities [30]. The potential for patients to meet with people in similar circumstances from the wider community to engage in physical activity can provide an opportunity to build relationships and a supportive solution to increase activity levels [31]. Social support is important for the adoption and maintenance of physical activity, particularly for older adults [32].

The role that healthcare professionals play in promoting physical activity as part of routine care, and the support that they provide for older adults will be increasingly important in addressing the fall-out from COVID-19 on older adult's health. It is likely that the proportion of the older adult population inactive and at risk from disease and disorders related to inactivity will have increased [33]. Those who are socio-economically disadvantaged, frail, living with multimorbidity or disability or living in residential care, may have been disproportionately affected [34].

Strengths and Limitations

This study captured views from a diverse range of healthcare professions. To the authors' knowledge, this is the first study to have completed this type of analysis across the island of Ireland. The TDF was utilised as an evidence-based method for identifying individual and organisational determinants of health professionals' behaviour and decision-making. In this context, questions used within the questionnaire had established content validity and extensive piloting and pre-development work, which with the input of an expert advisory group, improved the overall validity of the final survey. The questionnaire was distributed through professional body networks across the island of Ireland and the number of valid responses (conceivably affected by the COVID-19 pandemic, during which healthcare professionals were facing unprecedented demands on their time) compares favourably to other studies conducted with healthcare professionals. However, consideration should still be given to the generalisability of the survey findings. Selection bias is an issue that needs to be considered in this context, as it is possible that healthcare professionals who are interested in and utilise physical activity in routine practice were more motivated to participate. The smaller number of respondents from general practice and nursing (relative to physiotherapy and occupational therapy) is also a potential limitation of the research.

5. Conclusions

Healthcare professionals have a key role in the promotion of physical activity as part of a whole-systems approach. This is highlighted in the strategic objectives of National and International Policy.

This study has shown that healthcare professionals consider it a part of their role to discuss physical activity, and many reported that it was feasible to initiate discussions about physical activity even in the face of commonly reported barriers (little time available/patient not motivated).

Successful implementation of physical activity promotion in routine practice will have substantial health benefits at a population level, particularly for older adults who stand to benefit the most from increasing levels of activity. However, continuing education and training is essential to support healthcare professionals' knowledge and skill development if they are to be successful in this role.

Supplementary Materials: The following are available online at https://www.mdpi.com/article/10.3390/ijerph18116064/s1, Table S1: Theoretical domains of healthcare professionals' behaviour in assessment, discussion, and prescription of physical activity in routine practice.

Author Contributions: C.C. and R.O. were involved in the conception, design and methodology, administration, analysis, and writing—original draft preparation, review, and editing. Both authors have read and agreed to the published version of the manuscript.

Funding: This research received no external funding.

Institutional Review Board Statement: The study was conducted according to the guidelines of the Declaration of Helsinki and approved by an Independent Peer Review panel (Ref: 2020-03-HCP).

Informed Consent Statement: Informed consent was obtained from all subjects involved in the study.

Data Availability Statement: Data is contained within the article or supplementary material (Table S1).

Acknowledgments: The authors would like to acknowledge the support from members of the Research Project Advisory Group in pilot testing, refinement, approval, and promotion of the survey.

Conflicts of Interest: The authors declare no conflict of interest.

References

1. Cunningham, C.; Sullivan, R.O.; Caserotti, P.; Tully, M.A. Consequences of physical inactivity in older adults: A systematic review of reviews and meta-analyses. *Scand. J. Med. Sci. Sport.* **2020**, *30*, 816–827. [CrossRef] [PubMed]
2. Davies, D.S.C.; Atherton, F.; McBride, M.; Calderwood, C. UK Chief Medical Officers' Physical Activity Guidelines. Dep. Heal. Soc. Care, no. September; 2019; pp. 1–65. Available online: https://www.gov.uk/government/publications/physical-activity-guidelines-uk-chief-medical-officers-report (accessed on 15 April 2021).
3. *WHO Guidelines on Physical Activity and Sedentary Behaviour*; World Health Organization: Geneva, Switzerland, 2020.
4. Payette, H.; Gueye, N.R.; Gaudreau, P.; Morais, J.A.; Shatenstein, B.; Gray-Donald, K. Trajectories of physical function decline and psychological functioning: The Quebec longitudinal study on nutrition and successful aging (NuAge). *J. Gerontol. B. Psychol. Sci. Soc. Sci.* **2011**, *66*, 82–90. [CrossRef] [PubMed]
5. Cunningham, C.; O'Sullivan, R. Physical Activity and Older Adults. An Overview of Guidelines, Trends, Policies and Frameworks. Dublin, Ireland. 2019. Available online: https://www.publichealth.ie/document/iph-report/physical-activity-and-older-adults-overview-guidelines-trends-policies-and (accessed on 15 April 2021).
6. World Health Organization. More Active People for a Healthier World. *J. Policy Model.* **2018**, *28*, 615–627.
7. World Health Organization. *Integrating Diet, Physical Activity and Weight Management Services into Primary Care*; World Health Organization, Regional Office for Europe: Copenhagen, Denmark, 2016.
8. Wheeler, P.C.; Mitchell, R.; Ghaly, M.; Buxton, K. Primary care knowledge and beliefs about physical activity and health: A survey of primary healthcare team members. *BJGP Open* **2017**, *1*, 809. [CrossRef]
9. Jelley, S.; Lake, A. *Physical Activity: Brief Advice for Adults in Primary Care*; NICE: London, UK, 2013.
10. Thornton, J.S.; Frémont, P.; Khan, K.; Poirier, P.; Fowles, J.; Wells, G.D.; Frankovich, R.J. Physical Activity Prescription: A Critical Opportunity to Address a Modifiable Risk Factor for the Prevention and Management of Chronic Disease: A Position Statement by the Canadian Academy of Sport and Exercise Medicine. *Clin. J. Sport Med.* **2016**, *26*, 259–265. [CrossRef]
11. Health Service Executive. *Making Every Contact Count: A Health Behaviour Change Framework and Implementation Plan for Health Professionals in the Irish Health Service*; Health Service Executive: Dublin, Ireland, 2016.
12. Chatterjee, R.; Chapman, T.; Brannan, M.G.T.; Varney, J. GPs' knowledge, use, and confidence in national physical activity and health guidelines and tools: A questionnaire-based survey of general practice in England. *Br. J. Gen. Pract.* **2017**, *67*, e668–e675. [CrossRef]
13. Lowe, A.; Littlewood, C.; McLean, S.; Kilner, K. Physiotherapy and physical activity: A cross-sectional survey exploring physical activity promotion, knowledge of physical activity guidelines and the physical activity habits of UK physiotherapists. *BMJ Open Sport Exerc. Med.* **2017**, *3*, 1–7. [CrossRef]
14. Cuthill, J.A.; Shaw, M. Questionnaire survey assessing the leisure-time physical activity of hospital doctors and awareness of UK physical activity recommendations. *BMJ Open Sport Exerc. Med.* **2019**, *5*, e000534. [CrossRef]
15. Atkins, L.; Francis, J.; Islam, R.; O'Connor, D.; Patey, A.; Ivers, N.; Foy, R.; Duncan, E.M.; Colquhoun, H.; Grimshaw, J.M.; et al. A guide to using the Theoretical Domains Framework of behaviour change to investigate implementation problems. *Implement. Sci.* **2017**, *12*, 77. [CrossRef]
16. Norton, T.C.; Rodriguez, D.C.; Willems, S. Applying the Theoretical Domains Framework to understand knowledge broker decisions in selecting evidence for knowledge translation in low- and middle-income countries. *Health Res. Policy Syst.* **2019**, *17*, 1–15. [CrossRef]
17. Milton, K.; Bull, F.C.; Bauman, A. Reliability and validity testing of a single-item physical activity measure. *Br. J. Sports. Med.* **2011**, *45*, 203–208. [CrossRef]

18. Sallis, R.E.; Matuszak, J.M.; Baggish, A.L.; Franklin, B.A.; Chodzko-Zajko, W.; Fletcher, B.J.; Gregory, A.; Joy, E.; Matheson, G.; McBride, P.; et al. Call to action on making physical activity assessment and prescription a medical standard of care. *Curr. Sports Med. Rep.* **2016**, *15*, 207–214. [CrossRef] [PubMed]
19. Kime, N.; Pringle, A.; Zwolinsky, S.; Vishnubala, D. How prepared are healthcare professionals for delivering physical activity guidance to those with diabetes? A formative evaluation. *BMC Health Serv. Res.* **2020**, *20*, 1–12. [CrossRef]
20. Ojo, S.O.; Bailey, D.P.; Hewson, D.J.; Chater, A.M. Perceived barriers and facilitators to breaking up sitting time among desk-based office workers: A qualitative investigation using the TDF and COM-B. *Int. J. Environ. Res. Public Health* **2019**, *16*, 2903. [CrossRef] [PubMed]
21. Pears, S.; Bijker, M.; Morton, K.; Vasconcelos, J.; Parker, R.A.; Westgate, K.; Brage, S.; Wilson, E.; Prevost, A.T.; Kinmonth, A.L.; et al. A randomised controlled trial of three very brief interventions for physical activity in primary care. *BMC Public Health* **2016**, *16*, 1–13. [CrossRef] [PubMed]
22. Hardcastle, S.J.; Taylor, A.H.; Bailey, M.P.; Harley, R.A.; Hagger, M.S. Effectiveness of a motivational interviewing intervention on weight loss, physical activity and cardiovascular disease risk factors: A randomised controlled trial with a 12-month post-intervention follow-up. *Int. J. Behav. Nutr. Phys. Act.* **2013**, *10*, 1–17. [CrossRef]
23. O'Brien, S.; Prihodova, L.; Heffron, M.; Wright, P. Physical activity counselling in Ireland: A survey of doctors' knowledge, attitudes and self-reported practice. *BMJ Open Sport Exerc. Med.* **2019**, *5*, 1–10. [CrossRef]
24. Lawrence, W.; Watson, D.; Barker, H.; Vogel, C.; Rahman, E.; Barker, M. Meeting the UK Government's prevention agenda: Primary care practitioners can be trained in skills to prevent disease and support self-management. Perspect. *Public Health* **2021**, 1757913920977030. [CrossRef]
25. Pugh, G.; O'Halloran, P.; Blakey, L.; Leaver, H.; Angioi, M. Integrating physical activity promotion into UK medical school curricula: Testing the feasibility of an educational tool developed by the Faculty of Sports and Exercise Medicine. *BMJ Open Sport Exerc. Med.* **2020**, *6*, 1–6. [CrossRef]
26. Osborne, S.A.; Adams, J.M.; Fawkner, S.; Kelly, P.; Murray, A.D.; Oliver, C.W. Tomorrow's doctors want more teaching and training on physical activity for health. *Br. J. Sports Med.* **2017**, *51*, 624–625. [CrossRef]
27. Lobelo, F.; Rohm Young, D.; Sallis, R.; Garber, M.D.; Billinger, S.A.; Duperly, J.; Hutber, A.; Pate, R.R.; Thomas, R.J.; Widlansky, M.E.; et al. Routine Assessment and Promotion of Physical Activity in Healthcare Settings: A Scientific Statement From the American Heart Association. *Circulation* **2018**, *137*, e495–e522. [CrossRef]
28. Bowen, P.G.; Mankowski, R.T.; Harper, S.A.; Buford, T.W. Exercise is Medicine as a Vital Sign: Challenges and Opportunities. *Transl. J. Am. Coll. Sport. Med.* **2019**, *4*, 1–7. [CrossRef]
29. Carstairs, S.A.; Rogowsky, R.H.; Cunningham, K.B.; Sullivan, F.; Ozakinci, G. Connecting primary care patients to community-based physical activity: A qualitative study of health professional and patient views. *BJGP Open* **2020**, *4*, 1100. [CrossRef] [PubMed]
30. Matthews, A.; Jones, N.; Thomas, A.; van den Berg, P.; Foster, C. An education programme influencing health professionals to recommend exercise to their type 2 diabetes patients—Understanding the processes: A case study from Oxfordshire, UK. *BMC Health Serv. Res.* **2017**, *17*, 1–15. [CrossRef]
31. Tully, M.A.; Cunningham, C.; Cupples, M.E.; Farrell, D.; Hardeman, W.; Hunter, R.F.; Laventure, B.; McDonough, S.M.; Morgan, J.; Murphy, M.H.; et al. Walk with Me: A protocol for a pilot RCT of a peer-led walking programme to increase physical activity in inactive older adults. *Pilot Feasibility Stud.* **2018**, *4*, 1–12. [CrossRef]
32. Tully, M.A.; Cunningham, C.; Wright, A.; McMullan, I.; Doherty, J.; Collins, D.; Tudor-Locke, C.; Morgan, J.; Phair, G.; Laventure, B.; et al. Peer-led walking programme to increase physical activity in inactive 60- to 70-year-olds: Walk with Me pilot RCT. *Public Heal. Res.* **2019**, *7*, 1–124. [CrossRef] [PubMed]
33. Cunningham, C.; Sullivan, R.O. Why physical activity matters for older adults in a time of pandemic. *Eur. Rev. Aging Phys. Act.* **2020**, *17*, 17–20. [CrossRef] [PubMed]
34. Klempel, N.; Blackburn, N.E.; McMullan, I.L.; Wilson, J.J.; Smith, L.; Cunningham, C.; O'Sullivan, R.; Caserotti, P.; Tully, M.A. The effect of chair-based exercise on physical function in older adults: A systematic review and meta-analysis. *Int. J. Environ. Res. Public Health* **2021**, *18*, 1902. [CrossRef]

Article

Healthcare Professionals' Application and Integration of Physical Activity in Routine Practice with Older Adults: A Qualitative Study

Conor Cunningham [1,*] and Roger O'Sullivan [1,2]

1. Institute of Public Health, Belfast BT1 4JH, UK; roger.osullivan@publichealth.ie
2. Bamford Centre for Mental Health and Wellbeing, Ulster University, Belfast BT37 0QB, UK
* Correspondence: conor.cunningham@publichealth.ie

Abstract: Healthcare professionals (HCPs) have a key role in promoting physical activity, particularly among populations at greatest risk of poor health due to physical inactivity. This research explored HCPs' knowledge, decision making, and routine practice of physical activity promotion with older adults. Furthermore, it aimed to enhance our understanding of the supports that HCPs need to effectively promote physical activity in routine practice across a wide range of healthcare professions, settings, and sectors. Semi-structured online interviews were completed with HCPs between November 2020–March 2021. Data were first analysed by coding instances within the transcripts, mapping onto relevant Theoretical Domains Framework (TDF) domains utilising a deductive thematic analysis approach. The data were then analysed utilising an inductive approach to thematically generate explanatory subthemes within the identified domains. Participants (*n* = 63) included general practitioners (15.87%), occupational therapists (30.16%), physiotherapists (38.10%), and nurses (15.87%) from the island of Ireland (Ireland and Northern Ireland). Of those interviewed, 10 (15.87%) were male and 53 (84.13%) were female. Two thirds (65.08%) were HCPs practicing in Ireland. Domains and subthemes related to the application of physical activity, and emergent themes on developing practice to support the application and integration of physical activity in routine practice are discussed. HCPs identified that focused education, appropriate training, and access to tailored resources are all essential to support the promotion of physical activity in routine practice. For such supports to be effective, a 'cultural shift' is required in HCP training and health service provision to adopt the growing evidence base that physical activity promotion must be part of disease prevention and treatment in routine practice. HCPs highlighted a range of areas for service development to support them to promote physical activity. Further research is required to explore the feasibility of implementing these recommendations in routine practice.

Keywords: physical activity; healthcare professionals; older adults; theoretical domains framework; policy; behaviour change

1. Introduction

International guidelines recommend that all older adults (65+ years) should aim to do at least 150 min of moderate intensity or 75 min of vigorous intensity aerobic activity throughout the week, with muscle strengthening and multicomponent balance training on 2 or more days per week [1]. For older adults meeting international physical activity recommendations, there is a significant reduction in the risk of all-cause mortality, Alzheimer's disease, and incident depression [2]. In addition to recommending that all older adults should undertake regular physical activity, these guidelines also emphasise the benefits of even small increases in physical activity and less time spent sedentary throughout the day, prompting the "move more, sit less" message [1]. However, for many, ageing is defined by rapid declines in levels of physical activity, loss of mobility and functional independence, and premature morbidity [3]. This stage of life therefore represents an important period to promote physical activity to improve functions of daily living and slow progression of disease and disability [4].

Physical activity promotion has increasingly been recognised as a priority for public health supported by the development of policies and interventions [4]. These actions recognise that addressing inactivity requires a 'whole of society' approach, with action across different sectors [5]. Key strategic objectives of this 'systems-based' approach in the health sector are to implement and strengthen systems of patient assessment and counselling on increasing physical activity and reducing sedentary behaviour by appropriately trained healthcare professionals (HCPs) [5] and to enhance the provision of, and opportunities for, appropriately tailored programmes and services aimed at increasing physical activity in older adults [6].

HCPs are well placed to promote physical activity through both structured and opportunistic contact [7,8]. They serve as influential sources of information and guidance with a wide range and number of patients and frequently engage with those in most need of physical activity advice, e.g., people with type 2 diabetes, depression, joint and back pain [2,9]. Integrating physical activity counselling and referral as part of routine brief interventions in primary healthcare systems is identified as a 'best buy' in public health with proven effectiveness in decreasing the burden of non-communicable diseases and improving quality of life [2,10].

While the promotion of physical activity should be a core competence for all primary healthcare professionals [11], challenges exist, such as time constraints, perceived lack of patient engagement, and competing priorities [12]. In addition, there is a recognition of the need for greater teaching in this area at both undergraduate and postgraduate levels [12], and for the provision of additional in-service training and evidence-informed resources to support effective promotion of physical activity in routine practice [13]. Our own research in this area identified a need for continuing professional education and skill development [14], and while programmes have been introduced to develop knowledge of how to carry out a brief intervention with patients or service users, there is still a broad recognition of the need for further supports in this area to enable HCPs to effectively assess, counsel, and support their patients to increase levels of physical activity [14–16].

This research sought to develop our understanding of the supports (individual and structural/organisational) that HCPs need to effectively promote physical activity (through assessment, discussion, and prescription) in routine practice with older adults. Furthermore, this research aimed to enhance our understanding of knowledge (how it is developed and implemented in practice) and decision making (barriers/facilitators and models of good practice in physical activity promotion) in relation to physical activity promotion as part of routine care with older adults on the island of Ireland (Ireland and Northern Ireland).

2. Materials and Methods

This qualitative study was the third phase of a broad programme of research comprising a systematic review of reviews, a quantitative survey, and this qualitative follow-up. The systematic review of reviews (Phase 1) provided a comprehensive and systematic overview of epidemiological evidence from previously conducted research to assess the associations of physical activity with physical and mental health outcomes in older adults [2]. Phase 2 involved a cross-sectional survey of HCPs' knowledge and routine practice of physical activity promotion with older adults on the island of Ireland (Ireland and Northern Ireland) [14]. The purpose of this qualitative component (Phase 3) was to build on the survey findings to further enhance our understanding of HCPs' knowledge and decision making in relation to physical activity promotion and explore HCPs' own views on the supports that are needed to effectively apply and integrate physical activity promotion in routine practice across a wide range of healthcare professions, settings, and sectors.

2.1. Design and Sampling

This qualitative component used semi-structured, online interviews. Respondents (general practitioners, occupational therapists, nurses, and physiotherapists) from the previous survey (Phase 2) were asked if they consented to future contact from the research team [14]. Those who agreed were e-mailed an invitation to participate (including participant information sheet and consent form). Other participants were recruited through professional bodies for general practice, physiotherapy, nursing, and occupational therapy on the island of Ireland. A purposive sampling method was used to ensure that each profession was represented. Sampling continued until there was a consensus by the authors that theoretical and content saturation had occurred. A total of n = 63 HCPs participated (see Table 1). The study was conducted according to the guidelines of the Declaration of Helsinki and independently peer reviewed.

Table 1. Characteristics of interview participants.

	All Interviewees	
	N	%
Professional affiliation		
General practitioner	10	15.87
Physiotherapist	24	38.10
Occupational therapist	19	30.16
Nurse	10	15.87
Gender		
Male	10	15.87
Female	53	84.13
Years qualified		
0–5	2	3.17
6–10	10	15.87
11–15	12	19.05
16–20	20	31.75
21–25	8	12.70
26+	11	17.46
Healthcare setting		
Primary	44	69.84
Secondary	5	7.94
Other (e.g., residential)	14	22.22
Health sector		
Public	55	87.30
Private	7	11.11
Other	1	1.59
Region		
Northern Ireland	22	34.92
Ireland	41	65.08
Total	63	100

2.2. Data Collection

An interview schedule was developed and pilot tested by the research team based on the key theoretical domains explored in the survey which identified, in particular, the domains of Knowledge, Skills and Behavioural Regulation [14]. The schedule included questions on key topics related to national guidelines for physical activity for older adults; knowledge and practice of assessment/discussion/prescription of physical activity with patients as part of routine care; perceived opportunities to promote physical activity in day-to-day practice; the supports (individual and structural/organisational) that HCPs need to effectively promote physical activity (through assessment, discussion, and prescription) in routine practice, and questions related to implications of the COVID-19 pandemic on routine practice and views on the role of physical activity promotion to older adults in light of the pandemic. Analysis and findings of interview data related to the COVID-19 pandemic are reported in a separate publication.

Semi-structured interviews, lasting 30–45 min, were conducted by C.C. (who is experienced in qualitative methods), using an encrypted online phone service (Zoom) between November 2020–March 2021. Written and verbal informed consent was obtained prior to commencing the interview. Interviews were digitally recorded and coded audio files were transcribed verbatim. Any identifiable information was removed from coded transcripts.

2.3. Data Analysis

Data were analysed using NVivo software (version 12.0 Plus, QSR International, Melbourne, Australia). To establish an understanding of the application and integration of physical activity promotion in routine practice for HCPs, the data were first analysed by coding instances within the transcripts, mapping onto relevant Theoretical Domains Framework (TDF) domains [17], utilising a deductive thematic analysis approach. The 14-domain TDF is an integrative framework of theories of behaviour change which has been used to identify influences on HCP behaviour in the implementation of evidence-based recommendations [17] by analysing the social, environmental, cognitive, and affective influences on HCP practice [18]. The data were then analysed by utilising an inductive approach to thematically generate explanatory subthemes within the identified domains. One researcher (C.C.) conducted the coding of all transcripts, mapping of sub-themes, and data synthesis. A second researcher (R.O.) independently analysed a random sample of the interviews (20%). Any differences were discussed, and a consensus reached to ensure appropriateness of coding and mapping. The STROBE Checklist was used to guide the reporting of items to be included in reports of cross-sectional studies [19].

3. Results

A total of 63 individuals participated in the interviews, at which point no new emerging themes were identified. Participants included general practitioners (15.87%), occupational therapists (30.16%), physiotherapists (38.10%), and nurses (15.87%) from the island of Ireland. Participant characteristics are presented in Table 1. Of those interviewed, 10 (15.87%) were male and 53 (84.13%) were female. The majority of those interviewed had 16–20 years of practice experience (31.75%, $n = 20$). The proportion of those interviewed who reported that they worked in the public sector was 87.3% ($n = 55$) and two thirds (65.08%) were HCPs practicing in Ireland.

A summary of domains and subthemes related to knowledge of physical activity and application to routine practice, and area(s) for potential knowledge/practice development are presented in Table 2. Emergent themes on developing practice to support the application and integration of physical activity promotion are presented in Table 3. Additional HCP quotations coded during data analysis are presented in Supplementary Table S1.

In this section, we provide an overview of the emergent domains and subthemes from the analysis of interview data grouped under 'applying' and 'integrating' physical activity promotion to routine practice.

Table 2. Healthcare professionals' quotations for emergent domains and subthemes on application and integration (assessment/discussion/prescription) of physical activity in routine practice.

	TDF Domain	Subtheme	Exemplar Quotation	Area(s) Identified by HCPs for Potential Service Development
Applying physical activity to routine practice	Knowledge	Understanding health benefits	'There's good evidence that exercise, the strength and balance programmes, can significantly reduce falls, so there's a big payback there, in terms of preventing hip fractures' (NIGP1).	**Focused training** '... with my nursing background and my health promotion practice, they're really important messages for us to be sharing with the frontline staff, and then we have very strong evidence around the benefits of promoting health-enhancing physical activity to keep people active as they age, which will help to reduce their unhealthy weights and also reduce the risk of chronic conditions, or maybe delay the onset of chronic conditions...' (RoIN3).
		Source(s) of knowledge development	'I keep myself updated through the Public Health Agency, you know, anything that they would promote and publicise. And I try to link in with Councils and with my Health and Wellbeing Team, whenever it comes to them giving health promotion advice' (NIN2).	**Promoting (available) resources** 'So, I think obviously though, there is a lot out there that we can, you know, the use of apps and the NHS website now even, there's a lot of stuff to promote healthy lifestyle and there's a lot of free resources there. So, I am aware of those but I'm sure there's plenty I'm not aware of as well' (NIOT5).
		Initial and continuing professional development	'... since I qualified many years ago, all of my knowledge around guidelines, around activity would have been since graduation and it would have been from those courses' (NIN2).	**Education on behaviour change techniques** 'I think we need to be ... that whole psychology of it needs to be strengthened and developed more and that buying in and how we sell it ...' (RoIP3).
		Knowledge of physical activity guidelines	'I know the guidelines are there, am I up to date on them? Probably not but yeah, I obviously understand the importance of physical activity and make sure that that is brought into all treatments where feasible' (NIP1).	**Displaying Infographics** 'And as well then the government guidelines for physical activity, I wasn't totally aware of the exact recommendations of it until about two or three years ago. And those infographics now are everywhere in our department and everyone's very aware of the importance of physical activity, probably more so since then' (NIP4).
	Belief about consequences	Belief of the benefits for health	'... but I suppose we believe, I think that's the thing, I have no doubt of the benefits of exercise' (NIGP2).	

Table 2. Cont.

Social Professional Role and Identity	Social identity	'There is role modelling with it which I am quite keen to promote. Again, sometimes at lunch time I will go out running and I am quite keen that people recognise me as somebody who does that' (NIGP3).	**Health and wellbeing programmes for HCPs** 'I think there needs to be a bigger emphasis on health and wellbeing for staff before you'll probably see a huge knock-on effect for patients, or maybe you know concurrently even' (RoIP14).
	Professional identity	'And how important it is. And I think like when you're, yeah, it needs to be everyone's role definitely' (RoIOT3). 'Well I think it's everyone's realm' (NIP4).	**Reinforcing good practice that supports every HCP to promote physical activity** 'We would do in-service together and you know, have team meetings and we're always sort of asking what are you doing about this and how you're using this, what leaflets are you using, things like that. What outcome measures are you using? And like we all, in different areas had the falls prevention class and we were using that really well and everybody seemed to be enjoying it. So, from that point of view you know, we all seem to be doing the same thing' (NIP5).
	Organisational support for physical activity promotion	'So, we would have speech and language, we would have a dietician, we've nursing staff, physiotherapists, myself, OT and then once a week we have a geriatrician here as well which is brilliant, and then we have an SHO who's here every day as well. So, we're lucky you know, we're in a very good environment and we're very open and we're always open to trying different things. Like we had a wellness group here. We've done yoga before' (RoIOT2).	**Identifying supports for service delivery** So, in some of the areas we had a follow-on programme of 16 weeks, that was delivered again by [council service provider]. But not all areas within our trust had that. So, the Public Health Agency after I had brought that up, they fund the 16-week programme for all areas. I also said about the lack of weights, to be able to get the progressiveness with their exercises. And the Public Health Agency funded the weights (NIP6).
Skills	Assessing physical activity	'But I always say, 'What are your physical activity levels at the minute? What are your physical activity levels? What do you do?' They always say, 'I walk or play golf.' I always add it into the initial assessment or the chat with them' (NIP4).	**Formal assessment of physical activity** 'Yeah, I suppose we don't, in our team we don't really have a structure. It's something that probably needs to be put in place. Obviously in our assessment there will be, you know, previous mobility, it's basically as far as it goes' (NIP1).
Integrating physical activity promotion in routine practice: Assessment	Assessing functional status	So, generally, we do a comprehensive balance assessment initially. So, even if they're coming in with back pain, we still do a balance assessment with them to see where they are. We'd also do a bone health assessment with them. So, we obviously look at their bone health, particularly if they've had a recent fracture' (RoIP15).	

Table 2. Cont.

		Individual level (e.g., perception of patient motivation)	Motivational interview training (see below) and tailored support
		'And I'm trying to think ... yeah, we had another man who went home, but he was much, much less motivated, so that conversation would have been much shorter' (RoIP7).	'The barriers more are where people who say they physically can't do it. They say, "Oh, I have got a bad heart and I have bad knees." There is always some excuse, but we tailor the programmes to meet those needs as well and try to educate them a wee bit more in that they still can do light exercise and what are the health benefits for that. Most of them do try and do some sort of activities' (NIOT4).
	Barriers to physical activity promotion	Organisational (e.g., time)	Investing in prevention; Incentivising the use of physical activity in routine practice; Training and Practice Development and Service provision (see Table 3)
Environmental context and resources		'I think that's always been a big problem with GPs, is the lack of time you have with people for the lifestyle counselling and things' (NIGP5).	
		Societal (e.g., culture of physical activity)	Supportive Public Health Campaigns (see Table 3)
		'I just think ageing in Ireland has a different concept of itself, I don't think like, like I have obviously been on webinars where we've had Australians speaking and they talk about the older people over there having FitBits and going out walking, they're recording their steps and they're being very proactive about their exercise. Whereas I don't think that has filtered into Ireland or into the culture here yet' (RoIP5).	
	'Physical activity' or 'Exercise' as part of routine care		Focused Training in Clinical linguistics
		'I think people's eyes glaze over when the word exercise is mentioned. In a lot of places, it's actually not a very motivating word. So, I think certainly, physical activity, or broadening the scope of it, and the use of language, will help with motivating people' (RoIP2).	'At our [Professional body] conference this year, there was a guy giving a presentation on clinical linguistics, and the focus was on the language around pain. But a lot of the guidelines that he gave us would very much apply to motivating people in relation to physical activity. So, I think we probably have a lot of work to do still' (RoIP1).
Integrating physical activity promotion in routine practice: Discussion			
Memory, attention, and decision processes	Models of consultation		Motivational interview training
		'So, yes, I would say the vast majority of it is off my own experience and just probably reading the situation and learning from what I've done before in the past. So, yeah, yeah, no I can't really say I have formal teaching in that' (NIGP4).	'I would informally to myself go even with that approach and sort of chatting through on what's the person's goal and non-confrontational and rolling with resistance and all of that, even with that if the person is evidencing, they're just not interested' (RoIP7).

Table 2. Cont.

Integrating physical activity promotion in routine practice: Prescription	Environmental context and resources	Exercise is medicine	'But really, the more you hear about it, the more it's usually beneficial in management of so many conditions and the prevention of so many conditions' (NIGP4).
			Physical activity integrated into IT systems So, again, in our own software, it is individually, if I am putting in a blood pressure, I type in blood pressure and then temperature is a separate thing again. So, there isn't—I would have to look at exercise there. So, I don't think there is any formal exercise dialogue box there, if you like, as far as I know' (RoIGP5).
		Practice-based resource	'We also have a practice physio, but that would be more for people with specific orthopaedic conditions, back or knee pain, where you're sort of recommending specific exercises for that particular problem' (NIGP2).
			Supporting the development of innovative physical activity programmes 'So, then we trained up our own staff and we did like a walking group, we got that started and then we could pass over to the likes of [service provider]. We just kind of formed that bridge, tried to anyway in terms of physical activity' (NIP8).
		Social prescribing	'But there was social prescribing, you know, where you could refer to a local counsellor essentially, a local agent I suppose who knew what services were available in the area and can signpost people to what they needed' (NIGP4).
			Community resource mapping 'The biggest issue is that people know of pockets of good practice and people don't know what the landscape is so people don't know, we have no register or geographic map of what supports are out there or where you might tap into exercise' (RoIP10).
		Community-based resource	'[Name of Charity] have a tremendous exercise programme that we can refer patients as a referral, but patients can also contact themselves, which is walking clubs and gardening clubs and those sort of more normal physical activity, physical activity, but done in groups that stimulate people to make friendships and to keep it up more long-term' (NIGP1).
			Promoting community-practice linkage (see Table 3)

TDF: Theoretical Domains Framework; NIGP: Northern Ireland-based general practitioner; RoIGP: Ireland-based general practitioner; NIN: Northern Ireland-based nurse; RoIN: Ireland-based nurse; NIP: Northern Ireland-based physiotherapist; RoIP: Ireland-based physiotherapist; NIOT: Northern Ireland-based occupational therapist; RoIOT: Ireland-based occupational therapist.

Table 3. Healthcare professionals' quotations for emergent themes on developing practice to support the application and integration of physical activity promotion.

Area of Support Identified	Exemplar Quotation
Investing in prevention	'And so, if part of our role is to preserve life and the easiest way to do that and one of the cheapest ways is by promoting a healthy lifestyle ... So, it would be in the government's interest and in medical schools' interest and things like that to be putting funding and resources into those, into raising awareness' (RoIGP4).
Incentivising physical activity in routine practice	'I think money is just, I'm simplifying it, but I think that if you want to get, you know if the planners are saying, you know, moving, being active is going to be good for your health, it's going to be saving money in the long ... it's going to be good for people's health, which is the most important, but it's going to save money on hospitals, on medications down the line, well then we should invest in it, and if we're going to task professionals with promoting it, we should pay them' (RoIGP2).
Promoting community-practice linkage	In general practice ... 'Put the resources in a practice, like the MDT scheme, that helps them, that enables them. If you have a local resource, get them to come out to your practice and talk to you about it, rather than dumping them with a big bundle of papers' (NIGP3). In the acute setting ... '... like it would be great to have the knowledge about everything that's available in your catchment. But the reality is that that doesn't really happen, and a lot happens in the community that in the acute setting you're not aware of. Likewise, things happen in the acute setting that the community aren't aware of, I think it needs to be a bit broader than, you know, just limited to your own environment' (RoIN7).
Training development	In general practice (focused training) '... practical educational sessions that would be tailored to general practice, that would be based on the consultation. So, it would be a kind of a simulated workshop based on GP consultations, where you're basically demonstrating how this is done. A case-based simulation—active one-hour session that would be based locally for GPs and where GPs would be rewarded for going by getting CPD. Ultra-focused. It's not trying to do everything, and maybe the GP gets one skill and one practice-based tool out of it and no more' (RoIGP2). In Nursing (training and resource development in residential care) '... but some education, very practical, quick, easy, instructional maybe, multimedia, videos, laminated cards, about how we can introduce physical activity into everyday activities would be really, really helpful and I think it would be really beneficial to residents' physical and mental health' (RoIN6). In Physiotherapy ... '... good governance and clear training and ongoing CPD and you know, it's a challenging area. But I think it's a really needed area. And I think if you're looking to really you know, the gold standard and really improve, this is one really nice way of doing it' (RoIP3). For support staff (healthcare assistants) 'I think even general staff like healthcare assistants, particularly on a rehab ward. I think there should be some type of training for them, and I know there's staff pressures and stuff, but I think probably education would be a big thing and training for unqualified staff, to support with that gap in-between therapy' (NIOT5).
Practice development	'Yeah, so we need the service, so the health services to introduce physical activity competency as, I suppose, a quality indicator or an area, a specific area of work in health professionals' assessment in treatment of staff. So, it needs to be very explicit in terms of, you know, it being a core component of patient interventions, but we also need the professional bodies to actually, I suppose include it as a competency in terms of professional practice' (RoIN3). 'And I think if your standards and your compliance was measured those standards and that included how you integrate physical activity into the daily care that you deliver, and how you report on that in terms of your nursing documentation and your record keeping, I think that would go a long way to making sure that it became part and parcel of what we do' (RoIN6).

Table 3. Cont.

Area of Support Identified	Exemplar Quotation
Service provision	'I think unless there is more education, it will probably be like a status quo. I think it takes an education programme as to the importance of mobility. But unless they improve the staffing levels and improve the education, I think they could quite quickly be neglected' (NIN1).
Physical activity awareness campaign for staff (and public)	Supportive public health campaigns '... so you've got the public health champions and, you know, people, well-known sports stars promoting it and then you've got GPs on as well giving that message so that what the GP is doing is part of a greater movement for the good, and the GP is tying into it and it's natural and it feels easy and good and right to tie into that' (RoIGP2).

NIGP: Northern Ireland-based general practitioner; RoIGP: Ireland-based general practitioner; NIN: Northern Ireland- based nurse; RoIN: Ireland-based nurse; RoIP: Ireland-based physiotherapist; NIOT: Northern Ireland-based occupational therapist.

3.1. Applying Physical Activity to Routine Practice

At the beginning of each interview, HCPs were asked about their knowledge of physical activity guidelines in their jurisdiction, how and where they got their knowledge of physical activity and health, and how they felt this knowledge applied to routine practice.

3.2. TDF Domain: Knowledge

3.2.1. Emergent Subtheme: Knowledge and Understanding of the Benefits of Physical Activity for Patients' Health

There was a broad recognition of the benefits of physical activity for patients' health, across a range of both physical and mental health conditions that present in routine practice, and this was a consistent subtheme irrespective of healthcare setting, whether that be in the acute setting, in the community setting, or in residential care.

3.2.2. Emergent Subtheme: Source(s) of Knowledge Development

Several participants referred to current programmes designed to develop knowledge and application of brief interventions in routine practice (e.g., Making Every Contact Count), and more broadly, participants reported a wide range of sources to support their knowledge development. These represented: online resources, conferences, seminars, and webinars; professional bodies, societies, faculties, and associations; professional networks, and special interest groups (see Table 2).

3.2.3. Emergent Subtheme: Initial and Continuing Professional Education

Many HCPs acknowledged that their fundamental awareness of the role of physical activity in prevention and treatment of disease did not come from their undergraduate/initial education and training, and more specifically, that there is a need for continuing professional development (CPD) in relation to promoting physical activity for older adults' health. Many HCPs discussed how an interest in physical activity in general, and in the role that physical activity plays in health more specifically, had helped to define their continuing knowledge development.

3.2.4. Emergent Subtheme: Knowledge of Physical Activity Guidelines

Knowledge of physical activity guidelines varied considerably amongst HCPs. Some reported that they were aware of but could not recall specific components of the guidelines. Others reported that they utilise the guidelines daily and integrate them into every patient consultation (where appropriate). Most HCPs identified that using guidelines for physical activity in routine practice required a tailored approach, which followed initial discussions with a patient about their levels of physical activity or was contingent on their professional judgement and decision making in relation to how physical activity could be assessed, discussed, and prescribed with each patient.

3.3. TDF Domain: Belief about Consequences

Several HCPs cited their belief in the benefits of physical activity and exercise for both patients' health and their own health. For example,

> '... but I suppose we believe, I think that's the thing, I have no doubt of the benefits of exercise. And I even say it myself, even going back to my student days, I can remember people saying that they studied better when they were physically fitter. And I think there's ... so I think the whole mind and body thing, it helps both, is very true' (NIGP2).

3.4. TDF Domain: Social/Professional Role and Identity

3.4.1. Emergent Subtheme: Social Identity

Many HCPs acknowledged that being physically active (and being seen to be physically active) was a part of their social identity and that their perceived position of social influence and responsibility can be utilised to positively motivate patients to change behaviour.

3.4.2. Emergent Subtheme: Professional Identity

A subtheme that was consistently discussed was that promoting physical activity in routine practice should be a part of every HCP's job. Several HCPs identified that professional boundaries/roles (actual and perceived) may present a barrier to the application of physical activity to routine practice, and that there is potential for service development in some healthcare settings in addressing these barriers, so that all HCPs feel supported to apply physical activity to their routine patient care.

3.4.3. Emergent Subtheme: Organisational Support for Physical Activity Promotion

Several themes emerged from interviews related to actual and potential organisational (structural) support(s) for the application of physical activity in routine practice. For example, multi-disciplinary team (MDT) working was valuable to applying physical activity to routine practice. This was a consistent theme across healthcare settings, sectors, and regions (see Table 2 and Supplementary Table S1). Furthermore, a 'culture' of promoting physical activity at a departmental/organisational level was important to ensuring the effective application of physical activity promotion to routine practice. Several HCPs highlighted that there was still scope for improvement in addressing physical activity per se in comparison to other health promotion areas addressed in routine practice.

3.5. Integrating Physical Activity in Routine Practice

The emergent domains and subthemes for integrating physical activity promotion in routine practice are outlined and discussed below under patient assessment, discussions with patients about physical activity, and prescribing physical activity.

3.6. Patient Assessment

HCPs were asked about assessing levels of physical activity with patients in routine practice.

3.7. TDF Domain: Skill

3.7.1. Emergent Subtheme: Assessing Physical Activity as Part of Routine Practice

In general, assessing physical activity in routine practice, across all healthcare professions, followed an informal approach, relying on a conversation between HCP and patient to establish a patient's levels of physical activity, with several HCPs identifying the adoption of a more 'formal' assessment as an area for (potential) CPD. Assessing physical activity as a 'Vital Sign' was discussed. More specifically, general practitioners (GPs) identified this as a concept that could contribute to the promotion of physical activity in their routine practice.

3.7.2. Emergent Subtheme: Assessing Functional Status

Assessing functional status with patients was notably more structured, which may reflect the principle aims of restoring and management of functional status in falls prevention and preserving independence in activities of daily living that were discussed by many HCPs.

3.8. Discussions with Patients about Physical Activity

HCPs were asked how often they discussed physical activity with patients, how they initiated the conversation, and what were the barriers and facilitators to discussions about physical activity in routine practice.

3.9. TDF Domain: Memory, Attention, and Decision Processes
Emergent Subtheme: Models of Consultation

Several HCPs reported that they were guided by how the consultation unfolded, and the rapport that was developed with the patient during the consultation as to whether to discuss physical activity. Several discussed strategies to address common barriers that patients may put forward to not wanting to engage with physical activity and also discussed that routine promotion of physical activity was reinforced by positive patient feedback.

3.10. TDF Domain: Environmental Context and Resources
3.10.1. Emergent Subtheme: Barriers to Physical Activity Promotion in Routine Practice

A number of individual level (patient), organisational (waiting lists/caseloads/staff resource), and societal (cultural role of physical activity) level barriers were identified across the health professions to the routine integration of physical activity promotion in discussions with patients (See Table 2). For example, a patient's engagement (or perceived engagement) with physical activity promotion was identified as a potential barrier to the integration of physical activity in routine patient care.

A lack of time to routinely integrate physical activity in patient consultations, lengthy patient waiting lists, and large caseloads was a commonly cited theme. Limited resources (e.g., staffing levels) were also identified as barriers which impact the capacity of HCPs to effectively integrate physical activity promotion in routine care, and for older adults in particular, several HCPs identified that a barrier was the 'cultural' role that physical activity plays in the lives of many older adults on the island of Ireland (see Table 2).

3.10.2. Emergent Subtheme: 'Physical Activity' or 'Exercise' as Part of Routine Care

There was a general lack of clarity and consistency with the terms used interchangeably, and several HCPs identified the need to differentiate between the terms 'exercise' and 'physical activity' with patients as 'exercise' has potential negative connotations for some older adults. Several HCPs identified a need to develop the context for its use in discussions with patients in routine care, and several HCPs identified a need to address the correct use of terminology as a potential area for further CPD. One participant highlighted a professional body scheme (physiotherapy) which was developed to address this,

> '... there was a campaign over the last few years and it was about you know, 'hate exercise, love activity'. That exercise is not just for the people who go to the gyms and take part in triathlons, but it can be incorporated into life' (NIP2).

3.11. Prescribing Physical Activity

HCPs were asked about physical activity prescription, referral, and community practice linkage. As most interviews took place during the COVID-19 pandemic, participants were asked to reflect on 'typical' practice prior to the pandemic and reflect on their experiences of prescribing physical activity as part of routine practice.

3.12. TDF Domain: Environmental Context and Resources

3.12.1. Emergent Subtheme: Exercise Is Medicine

The theme that 'exercise is medicine' arose in several interviews with HCPs, with the discussions typically involving the role that both the individual and the wider community can take in promoting physical activity to improve health.

3.12.2. Emergent Subtheme: Practice-Based Resource

The MDT structure was highlighted as important for both integrating physical activity in routine care and for promoting community-practice linkage.

3.12.3. Emergent Subtheme: Social Prescribing

The importance of having a 'community navigator', either within the structure of the MDT, as part of the wider integrated care partnership or embedded in the community was highlighted in several interviews as important for the integration of physical activity in routine care, with one HCP highlighting a networking opportunity as a potential mechanism to facilitate knowledge translation of service provision at a community level (see Supplementary Table S1).

3.12.4. Emergent Subtheme: Community-Based Resource

The range and availability of community-based resources for HCPs to refer into was highlighted as a significant facilitator in integrating physical activity in routine care, whether that referral was to another community-based HCP, or to an established community-based programme run by a range of providers that had sufficient and appropriate structures in place to support patients. It was highlighted frequently that a well-developed and resourced program can have significant benefits for increasing participation in older adults, for example,

> 'We were told that older people wouldn't come in for the exercise class. We were told they just don't do it. And I think by the end of our last class, we would have run three classes over a week and had 45 patients in' (RoIP15).

However, it was also clear that the range and availability of community-based resource(s) varied considerably between practices and communities, from state-of-the-art facilities to little or no access to onward referral.

3.13. Developing Practice to Support the Application and Integration of Physical Activity Promotion

Several areas for potential service development were highlighted that could support HCPs to integrate (or further integrate) physical activity into routine practice. HCPs' quotations for emergent themes on developing practice to support the application and integration of physical activity promotion are presented in Table 3.

4. Discussion

Current evidence suggests that appropriate education, training, and access to resources are essential for supporting promotion of physical activity in routine practice for older adults [14]. This research sought to explore these themes in detail and adds HCPs' own views on the supports that are needed to effectively apply and integrate physical activity promotion in routine practice. It explores these concepts across a wide range of healthcare professions, settings and sectors, and aligns emergent themes to key theoretical domains of HCPs' behaviour to further our understanding of this area.

The key findings from this research confirm that focused education, appropriate training, and access to tailored resources are all essential to support the promotion of physical activity in routine practice. In addition, this research highlights that for these supports to be effective, a 'cultural shift' is required in HCP training and health service provision to adopt the routine application and integration of physical activity promotion in the health services.

4.1. Applying Physical Activity to Routine Practice

Many HCPs in this study highlighted continuing education and skill development as essential to raise their confidence and competence to undertake assessment and provide brief advice and/or counselling on physical activity in routine practice with older adults. Many accredited their 'working' knowledge of physical activity in prevention and treatment to continuing professional development rather than to their undergraduate/initial education and training. This is consistent with previous research that has highlighted the need for postgraduate training for HCPs to effectively address health behaviour change in routine care [20] and highlights the need for continuing support in the development and maintenance of programmes and interventions that facilitate HCPs continuing knowledge development.

4.2. TDF Domain: Knowledge

Four subthemes emerged under the TDF domain of 'Knowledge' (see Table 2). Discussions with HCPs consistently turned to the need for increased service provision of training and practice development to support knowledge development of the application of physical activity in routine practice with older adults. Increasing continuing professional 'knowledge' development is particularly important given that recent research has highlighted that HCPs' knowledge of physical activity guidelines varies considerably across healthcare professions and that having a detailed knowledge and recall of physical activity guidelines was associated with formal assessment, initiating discussion, and referral/signposting to physical activity services as part of routine practice [14]. In this research many HCPs also identified that there was still scope for improvement in addressing physical activity in comparison to other health promotion areas addressed in routine practice with older adults. Previous research suggests that HCPs consider physical activity to be less important than other health promotion activities such as smoking cessation [21]. In this research HCPs identified 'focused training'; 'promoting available resources'; 'education on behaviour change techniques' and 'displaying infographics' as potential areas for service development to promote HCPs' knowledge development of the application of physical activity to routine practice (See Tables 2 and 3).

4.3. TDF Domains: Social/Professional Role and Identity

HCPs also highlighted that knowledge development impacts on a HCPs 'professional identity': the set of behaviours and displayed personal qualities of an individual in a work setting (TDF domain: Social/Professional role and identity) [17]. Several HCPs identified that professional boundaries/roles (actual and perceived) can affect their confidence to apply physical activity to routine practice. Indeed, a recent study among nursing students in Ireland highlighted a lack of confidence in physical activity and recommended the integration of more physical activity education into the nursing curriculum to equip the future nursing workforce with the skills and confidence they need to promote physical activity to their patients [22]. Several participants identified MDT working as a model of good practice that facilitates the application of physical activity to routine care of older adults by removing potential role-related barriers. It was suggested that integrated models of practice also helped to establish a 'culture' where every HCP works effectively together to 'share' knowledge and apply physical activity to a patient's care.

Changing the 'culture' of health services to apply physical activity promotion as part of disease prevention requires leadership throughout organisational structures, and clinical leadership is essential in demonstrating support for the development of programmes and services that have the potential to reduce the burden of chronic disease [20]. The current Making Every Contact Count (MECC) program, to provide training in brief (and opportunistic) interventions to all healthcare professionals who may have patient contact in Ireland and Northern Ireland has highlighted the need for a long-term commitment to training support of HCPs in this role, and the need to reach a critical mass of trained staff to implement this agenda [20].

4.4. TDF Domain: Belief about Consequences

Several HCPs cited their belief in the benefits of physical activity for both older patients and their own health, and that continuing professional development in this respect was central to embedding physical activity in their routine practice. It also impacted on their 'social identity', with several of those interviewed (particularly GPs) highlighting that they were keen to been seen to 'practice what they preach'. 'Health and wellbeing programmes' for HCPs was identified as an area for potential service development to foster knowledge and subsequent belief of the benefits of physical activity that may transition into routine practice. The national physical activity plan for Ireland highlights the pivotal role that HCPs play in promoting physical activity and that they should be supported to lead more active lives through supportive workplace practices and policies [23]. Indeed, research suggests that clinicians who are physically active themselves are more likely to counsel patients about physical activity in routine care and may serve as a more convincing role model to their patients [24].

4.5. Integrating Physical Activity Promotion in Routine Practice

In addition to applying physical activity to routine practice, HCPs were asked about integrating physical activity promotion into routine practice. The emergent domains and subthemes for integrating physical activity promotion in routine practice are outlined and discussed under 'patient assessment', 'discussions with patients about physical activity' and 'prescribing physical activity'.

4.6. Patient Assessment: TDF Domain: Skills

The assessment of physical activity levels by HCPs in routine practice is the cornerstone of the counselling process [24] and is a key action recommended by the WHO to promote health-enhancing physical activity. In this study, 'formal' assessment of physical activity as part of routine practice was identified as an area of potential service development across all health professions, but particularly in general practice where it could be supported through integration in electronic medical records (EMR)/IT systems. Embedding physical activity as a 'vital sign' in EMR with 'pop-ups' to prompt the assessment of physical activity is both feasible and effective but requires training, appropriate infrastructure, and incentive to effectively integrate into models of patient consultation [24].

Several barriers were identified by HCPs in integrating physical activity assessment in routine practice with older adults, including 'time' and 'lack of incentive'. These barriers are reported widely within the literature [25]. Previous research has also highlighted that the lack of formal assessment in routine practice may reflect the level of training and support that HCPs have received on physical activity promotion broadly, and on physical assessment more specifically [14]. Nonetheless, many HCPs in this study identified that physical activity assessment should be standard practice in every patient consultation due to the numerous physical and mental health benefits for patients. It was felt that such future programmes and interventions that promote physical activity in the health services should contain appropriate and standardised training on physical activity assessment as part of routine care.

4.7. Discussions with Patients: TDF Domain: Memory, Attention, and Decision Processes

HCPs acknowledged that they are widely respected and trusted, and as such they have considerable potential to influence public and individual opinion, but they also reported that they face challenges in discussing physical activity with patients, namely 'time pressures' and 'caseloads'. HCPs also reported that their perception of an older patient's motivation to receive advice or discuss physical activity was an important component in decision making as to whether to initiate a discussion about physical activity. 'Motivational interview training' in the emergent subtheme 'Models of consultation' (TDF domain: Memory, attention, and decision processes) was highlighted as a potential area for practice development to support HCPs to anticipate barriers (such as patient motivation) and discuss patient-centred solutions to effectively address these barriers. Further to this, 'Education on behaviour change techniques' was also identified as a necessary component of initial and continuing professional education (TDF Domain: Knowledge). Evidence demonstrates the increased effect of brief physical activity interventions that use valid (and multiple) behaviour change methods, namely, behavioural, cognitive, and motivational approaches [7].

4.8. TDF Domain: Environmental Context and Resources

HCPs also highlighted several 'organisational' and 'societal' barriers to the routine integration of physical activity in discussions with patients, and this was consistent across professions and healthcare settings. Several participants identified that greater 'Investing in prevention' was required to adequately fund training and resources to support HCPs to effectively integrate physical activity promotion into routine practice and to move away from a 'treatment' model of healthcare to 'prevention', but to support this, campaigns are required to raise both HCPs and the general public's awareness of the benefits of physical activity through 'Supportive public health campaigns'. Public education campaigns that involve mass, digital and social media, outdoor billboards and posters, and mass distribution of information are an effective way to transmit consistent and clear messages about physical activity to a large population, and have been highlighted as one of eight investments that 'work' for physical activity in a call to action for embedding physical activity in national and subnational policies [10].

4.9. Prescribing Physical Activity: TDF Domain: Environmental Context and Resources

Prescribing 'exercise as medicine' and signposting older adult patients to physical activity services (i.e., exercise referral programmes/community-based physical activity initiatives) in routine practice has been shown to be associated with a detailed knowledge of the application of physical activity to routine care [14]. How the topic is raised and linked to a patient's specific health conditions is central to patient acceptance to the topic [13]. Research also suggests that the 'motivation' provided by HCPs is key to whether a patient accepts offers of being signposted to community physical activity opportunities [26,27], highlighting again the need for specific and ongoing education and training on exercise prescription as part of routine care. In this study, several participants discussed models of good practice in implementing referral pathways from both primary and acute care to community- or university-based programmes. They described how these models can provide that 'motivation' to patients through continuing care and support, tailored to their needs, in a local community setting with programmes that provide the key techniques for behaviour change (e.g., goal setting and social support) that are essential to the adoption and maintenance of a more physically active lifestyle [28].

It was clear in interviews with HCPs, however, that these models of referral were 'pockets' of good practice and, in general, there was significant variability in access to and availability of community-based resources across settings and professions. Previous research on the requirements for community-based provision has consistently highlighted the need for better community-based collaborations with sport, leisure, and fitness providers, but also improvements in infrastructure to support physical activity behaviour change [25]. In this study, in-service support through resource allocation and funding was highlighted as necessary in 'supporting the development of innovative physical activity programmes' whereas those HCPS who had shown initiative and developed a service to link community and practice have received retrospective health system funding to maintain that service (see Table 2).

Multi-disciplinary team working also facilitated patient referral utilising the available HCP resource within a practice. HCPs who worked in a setting that had access to a social prescriber also identified this as an extremely valuable resource, highlighting that this individual or service was key to the development and maintenance of effective community-practice linkage through 'community resource mapping' (see Table 3). A framework for the integration and mainstreaming of social prescribing within the health service in Ireland has recently been published [29].

4.10. Strengths and Limitations

This study captured views from a diverse range of healthcare professions and the TDF was utilised as an evidence-based method for identifying determinants of HCPs' application and integration of physical activity promotion in routine practice. It involved 63 interviews across two jurisdictions and two different healthcare systems. However, consideration should still be given to the generalisability of the study findings. Selection bias is an issue that needs to be considered in this context, as it is possible that HCPs who are interested in and utilise physical activity in routine practice were more motivated to participate. The smaller number of respondents from general practice and nursing (relative to physiotherapy and occupational therapy), and the predominately female sample is also a potential limitation of the research. However, the overall patterns of participation in this study are consistent with other studies conducted in this area and reflect the gender profile of the four professions.

5. Conclusions

Irrespective of profession, focused education, appropriate training, and access to tailored resources are all essential to support the promotion of physical activity in routine practice. However, it is evident that for such supports to be effective, a 'cultural shift' is required in HCP training and health service provision to adopt the growing evidence base that physical activity promotion must be part of disease prevention and treatment in routine practice.

Support programmes and campaigns to develop wider societal knowledge of the role of physical activity in health must be part of this process. There needs to be a shift in age-based assumptions around physical activity that challenge both the HCP and the older person themselves about what is possible and beneficial as we grow older. However, at the core is the need for service and practice development to support the routine application and integration of physical activity promotion in the health services.

Further research is required to explore the feasibility of implementing the recommendations by HCPs on the application and integration of physical activity promotion in routine practice.

Supplementary Materials: The following are available online at https://www.mdpi.com/article/10.3390/ijerph182111222/s1, Table S1: Additional healthcare professionals' quotations for emergent domains and subthemes on the application and integration (assessment/discussion/prescription) of physical activity in routine practice.

Author Contributions: C.C. and R.O. were involved in the conception, design and methodology, administration, analysis, and writing—original draft preparation, review, and editing. All authors have read and agreed to the published version of the manuscript.

Funding: This research received no external funding.

Institutional Review Board Statement: The study was conducted according to the guidelines of the Declaration of Helsinki and approved by an Independent Peer Review panel (Ref: 2020-03-HCP).

Informed Consent Statement: Informed consent was obtained from all subjects involved in the study.

Data Availability Statement: Data is contained within the article or Supplementary Material Table S1.

Acknowledgments: The authors would like to acknowledge the support given to the research project from members of the Research Project Advisory Group.

Conflicts of Interest: The authors declare no conflict of interest.

References

1. World Health Organization. *Guidelines on Physical Activity and Sedentary Behaviour*; World Health Organization: Geneva, Switzerland, 2020.
2. Cunningham, C.; O'Sullivan, R.; Caserotti, P.; Tully, M.A. Consequences of physical inactivity in older adults: A systematic review of reviews and meta-analyses. *Scand. J. Med. Sci. Sports* **2020**, *30*, 816–827. [CrossRef]
3. Payette, H.; Gueye, N.R.; Gaudreau, P.; Morais, J.A.; Shatenstein, B.; Gray-Donald, K. Trajectories of physical function decline and psychological functioning: The Quebec longitudinal study on nutrition and successful aging (NuAge). *J. Gerontol. B Psychol. Sci. Soc. Sci.* **2011**, *66*, 82–90. [CrossRef] [PubMed]
4. Cunningham, C.; O'Sullivan, R. Physical Activity and Older Adults. An Overview of Guidelines, Trends, Policies and Frameworks. Dublin, Ireland. 2019. Available online: https://publichealth.ie/physical-activity-and-older-adults-an-overview-of-guidelines-trends-policies-and-frameworks/ (accessed on 20 June 2021).
5. World Health Organization. *Global Action Plan on Physical Activity 2018–2030: More Active People for a Healthier World*; World Health Organization: Geneva, Switzerland, 2018.
6. World Health Organization. *Integrating Diet, Physical Activity and Weight Management Services into Primary Care*; World Health Organization, Regional Office for Europe: Copenhagen, Denmark, 2016.
7. Pears, S.; Bijker, M.; Morton, K.; Vasconcelos, J.; Parker, R.A.; Westgate, K.; Brage, S.; Wilson, E.; Prevost, A.T.; Kinmonth, A.L.; et al. A randomised controlled trial of three very brief interventions for physical activity in primary care. *BMC Public Health* **2016**, *16*, 1033. [CrossRef] [PubMed]
8. Mendes, R.; Nunes Silva, M.; Santos Silva, C.; Marques, A.; Godinho, C.; Tomás, R.; Agostinho, M.; Madeira, S.; Rebelo-Marques, A.; Martins, H.; et al. Physical activity promotion tools in the portuguese primary health care: An implementation research. *Int. J. Environ. Res. Public Health* **2020**, *17*, 815. [CrossRef] [PubMed]
9. National Institute for Clinical Excellence (NICE). *Physical Activity: Brief Advice for Adults in Primary Care*; NICE: London, UK, 2013.
10. International Society for Physical Activity and Health (ISPAH). ISPAH's Eight Investments that Work for Physical Activity. November 2020. Available online: www.ISPAH.org/Resources (accessed on 9 August 2021).
11. World Health Organization. *Physical Activity Strategy for the WHO European Region. 2016–2025*; World Health Organization, Regional Office for Europe: Copenhagen, Denmark, 2015.
12. O'Brien, S.; Prihodova, L.; Heffron, M.; Wright, P. Physical activity counselling in Ireland: A survey of doctors' knowledge, attitudes and self-reported practice. *BMJ Open Sport Exerc. Med.* **2019**, *5*, 1–10. [CrossRef] [PubMed]
13. Carstairs, S.A.; Rogowsky, R.H.; Cunningham, K.B.; Sullivan, F.; Ozakinci, G. Connecting primary care patients to community-based physical activity: A qualitative study of health professional and patient views. *BJGP Open* **2020**, *4*, 1100. [CrossRef]
14. Cunningham, C.; O'Sullivan, R. Healthcare Professionals Promotion of Physical Activity with Older Adults: A Survey of Knowledge and Routine Practice. *Int. J. Environ. Res. Public Health* **2021**, *18*, 6064. [CrossRef]
15. Lowe, A.; Littlewood, C.; McLean, S.; Kilner, K. Physiotherapy and physical activity: A cross-sectional survey exploring physical activity promotion, knowledge of physical activity guidelines and the physical activity habits of UK physiotherapists. *BMJ Open Sport Exerc. Med.* **2017**, *3*, 1–7. [CrossRef]
16. Chatterjee, R.; Chapman, T.; Brannan, M.G.T.; Varney, J. GPs' knowledge, use, and confidence in national physical activity and health guidelines and tools: A questionnaire-based survey of general practice in England. *Br. J. Gen. Pract.* **2017**, *67*, e668–e675. [CrossRef]
17. Cane, J.; O'Connor, D.; Michie, S. Validation of the theoretical framework for use in behaviour change and implementation research. *Implement. Sci.* **2012**, *7*, 37. [CrossRef]
18. Atkins, L.; Francis, J.; Islam, R.; O'Connor, D.; Patey, A.; Ivers, N.; Foy, R.; Duncan, E.M.; Colquhoun, H.; Grimshaw, J.M.; et al. A guide to using the Theoretical Domains Framework of behaviour change to investigate implementation problems. *Implement. Sci.* **2017**, *12*, 77. [CrossRef]
19. von Elm, E.; Altman, D.G.; Egger, M.; Pocock, S.J.; Gøtzsche, P.C.; Vandenbroucke, J.P. The Strengthening the Reporting of Observational Studies in Epidemiology (STROBE) statement: Guidelines for reporting observational studies. *J. Clin. Epidemiol.* **2008**, *61*, 344–349. [CrossRef]
20. Health Service Executive. *Making Every Contact Count: A Health Behaviour Change Framework and Implementation Plan for Health Professionals in the Irish Health Service*; Health Service Executive: Dublin, Ireland, 2016.
21. Netherway, J.; Smith, B.; Monforte, J. Training Healthcare Professionals on How to Promote Physical Activity in the UK: A Scoping Review of Current Trends and Future Opportunities. *Int. J. Environ. Res. Public Health* **2021**, *18*, 6701. [CrossRef]
22. Walsh, L.M.; Callaghan, H.P.; Keaver, L.M. Physical activity knowledge, attitudes and behaviours among Irish nursing students. *Int. J. Health Promot. Educ.* **2021**, *59*, 145–155. [CrossRef]
23. Department of Health and the Department of Transport Tourism and Sport. *Get Ireland Active: The National Physical Activity Plan for Ireland. Department of Health and the Department of Transport. Tourism and Sport*; Department of Health and the Department of Transport Tourism and Sport: Dublin, Ireland, 2016.
24. Bowen, P.G.; Mankowski, R.T.; Harper, S.A.; Buford, T.W. Exercise is Medicine as a Vital Sign: Challenges and Opportunities. *Transl. J. Am. Coll. Sports Med.* **2019**, *4*, 1–7. [CrossRef]

25. Lobelo, F.; Rohm Young, D.; Sallis, R.; Garber, M.D.; Billinger, S.A.; Duperly, J.; Hutber, A.; Pate, R.R.; Thomas, R.J.; Widlansky, M.E.; et al. Routine Assessment and Promotion of Physical Activity in Healthcare Settings: A Scientific Statement from the American Heart Association. *Circulation* **2018**, *137*, e495–e522. [CrossRef] [PubMed]
26. Brannan, M.; Bernardotto, M.; Clarke, N.; Varney, J. Moving healthcare professionals -a whole system approach to embed physical activity in clinical practice. *BMC Med. Educ.* **2019**, *19*, 84. [CrossRef] [PubMed]
27. Matthews, A.; Jones, N.; Thomas, A.; Van Den Berg, P.; Foster, C. An education programme influencing health professionals to recommend exercise to their type 2 diabetes patients—Understanding the processes: A case study from Oxfordshire, UK. *BMC Health Serv. Res.* **2017**, *17*, 1–15. [CrossRef] [PubMed]
28. Tully, M.A.; Cunningham, C.; Wright, A.; McMullan, I.; Doherty, J.; Collins, D.; Tudor-Locke, C.; Morgan, J.; Phair, G.; Laventure, B.; et al. Peer-led walking programme to increase physical activity in inactive 60- to 70-year-olds: Walk with Me pilot RCT. *Public Health Res.* **2019**, *7*, 1–124. [CrossRef] [PubMed]
29. Health Service Executive: Social Prescribing Framework. *Mainstreaming Social Prescribing in Partnership with Community & Volunatry Organisations*; Health Service Executive: Dublin, Ireland, 2021. Available online: https://www.drugsandalcohol.ie/34592/ (accessed on 6 September 2021).

Article
Onset of Weight Gain and Health Concerns for Men: Findings from the TAP Programme

Mark Cortnage [1,*] and Andy Pringle [2]

1. School Allied and Public Health, Anglia Ruskin University, Young Street, Cambridge CB1 2LZ, UK
2. Human Sciences Research Centre, University of Derby, Kedleston Road, Derby DE22 1GB, UK; a.pringle@derby.ac.uk
* Correspondence: mark.cortnage@aru.ac.uk

Abstract: With shown reticence by men to engage with dietary interventions for weight loss, investigations that provide detail on men's perceptions for the causes of weight gain and subsequent concerns over health and image are important. Such discoveries have potential to make a valuable contribution to male gendered programme design aimed at tackling weight gain and promoting good health. Connecting to men to health using their hobbies and interests, this study deployed semi-structured interviews of eight male participants (age > 35 years) enrolled on The Alpha Programme (TAP). TAP is a 12-week football and weight management intervention delivered in local community venues. Results captured men's lived experiences and feelings of being overweight, their attempts at dietary modification, health and causes of weight gain. Results signify externalized attribution for weight gain, entrenched habitual intake practices, despondency related to weight stigmatization, self-objectification and low self-worth. Moreover, this study outlines the processes for capturing this information using a male friendly approach and setting. Outcomes have potential for shaping bespoke men's weight management and health improvement interventions in the future.

Keywords: obesity; football; weight gain; sedentary; weight stigmatization; physical activity; self-esteem; men; self-objectification

1. Introduction

Feelings of being overweight and obese have limited research coverage. Recognising the low engagement with health services, men may not consider incentives such as dieting and health improvement as strong motivators to tackle weight, whereas alternative incentives may be more enticing, namely opportunities to improve performance and effectiveness [1]. Complementing insight into male perceived barriers to weight loss, by understanding perceptions of weight and the contribution of dietary related behaviours would help shape behavioural approaches accordingly.

Traditional masculine norms negatively ascribe help seeking behaviour with weakness, loss of control and autonomy [2,3]. For men to seek help risks stigmatisation [4] that if internalised can lead to further feelings of negativity towards counselling [3]. Although younger men are more inclined to engage in 'performative acts' such as risk taking, violence and excessive drinking [5], older men, perceived to be more risk adverse [6,7] portray a cautious appreciation of risk where age related decline in strength, fitness and sexual prowess manifest into efforts to halt said decline [8]. Yet, despite this perception, older male, health positive practice is not replicated in the UK data which underlines a persistent increase over the last 28 years of male overweight/obesity, rising from 58% of the total UK male population in 1993 to 68% in 2019 [9]. Across the age range 45 to 74 years 79% of the UK male population are either overweight or obese. UK males have increased mortality from avoidable disease than women at 150.2 deaths per 1000 (n = 3896) and 97.4 per 1000 (n = 2705) in 2019, respectively. Since 2011, the greatest slowdown in mortality improvement for men is ischaemic heart disease [10].

Stigmatisation has been associated with externalisation of identity, outlining self-objectification, e.g., ugly, horrible [11], often facilitating a degradation in emotional wellbeing [12,13]. In men Lozano et al. (2016) [14] found that weight stigma undermines men's sense of self-concept and men's masculine values and becomes a social threat—real or imagined—that entails negative psychosocial outcomes, preventing men's participation in social activities, including weight loss. Habitual unhealthy eating practices are capable of weakening self-efficacy to the point of undermining the effectiveness of commonly recommended dietary methods, e.g., planning and self-monitoring [15]. By exposing the thoughts of respondents as to the cause(s) of their weight gain, we can tailor more effective intervention.

A male study sample (n = 35) ages 35 to 64 years participated in a 91 week, optimised gendered football and nutrition programme named The Alpha Programme (TAP) which targeted weight loss as an empirically evaluated outcome. Qualitative feedback obtained from interviews was used to compare outcomes and evaluate the success of the intervention and identify key implementation considerations. These lived experiences are presented through themes identified related to health, weight, and diet.

For this programme, development of the Community of Practice (COP) [16] is facilitated through shared common interest, namely football. Knowledge exchange, shared experiences and personal development are particularly important to men who commonly display tendencies for social isolation, degraded mental health state and subsequent reduced health service engagement [17]. When coupled with stigmatisation in relation to weight we portray a demographic that may engage with health incentives through a conducive environment populated by likeminded individuals with a firm, yet empathetic Transformation Leadership [18].

2. Materials and Methods

2.1. Intervention Context

The Alpha Programme (TAP) was conceived in 2013 based on both empirical and research outlining the reluctance of men to access health services and engage with effective weight management incentives [19–21] with the aim of offering an innovative male gendered alternative to weight loss and management. TAP commenced on the 25 July 2015. Initial interviews were conducted during this week. The programme ran for a period of 91 weeks, considerably longer than the initial plan of 12 weeks. TAP achieved significant weight loss and maintenance at 91 weeks.

2.2. Ethical Consideration

Ethical principles 1 to 6 of the Economic and Social Research Council [22] were adhered to in all methods used in this study. The protocol outline was explained to the participants during the induction interview and participants were free to ask for clarification at any time. Stage 1 Ethical approval was sought from the Anglia Ruskin University Faculty Research Ethics Panel on a single occasion. Approval was accepted from the date 23rd June 2015 for three years. Reference Number: 15/026.

This research followed the best ethical guiding principles, specifically related to weight management programmes at the time. Research ethics in practice were aligned with Have al., (2013) "Ethical framework for the prevention of overweight and obesity" [23].

2.3. Instrumentation

The study utilised a convenience sampling method, a form of non-probability or non-random sampling where the sample were required to meet certain criteria, such as accessibility, proximity to the research and convenience [24], to recruit as many men as possible onto the programme.

For recruitment, leaflets were left at the reception of the football ground where the sessions were to be held. Leaflets were also divided between the researcher and volunteer coach who distributed to friends and acquaintances. Potential participants were able to contact the researcher directly via the contact details on the leaflet, register for attendance in person through the researcher or coach or register their interest at the football venue.

All participants completed an induction session consisting of a presentation prior to commencement of training. The presentation was followed by the completion of documents; two Participant Consent Forms (PCF) and one Participant Information Sheet (PIS). Alongside written details outlined in the PIS, further information about the study was presented to all participants during induction. The opportunity to ask (and address) questions continued throughout the session. Upon acceptance of the details included on the consent form and research protocol, recruits were asked to sign two copies of the PCF, with one copy handed back to the participant and the other retained by the researcher. All participants were provided with the PIF and encouraged to retain it.

Interviews are regularly used to investigate participants. In this study, interviews were voice recorded to help improve transcription accuracy. Each interview was digitally recorded using an Olympus WS-832 digital voice recorder. A further backup digital recorder, the Olympus DS-40 was used simultaneously in case of failure. Interviews were recorded in MP3 format and uploaded onto an online secure drive after recording. Recordings were transcribed against each question asked, with respondents identified by initials to protect anonymity. A quality control check was conducted, playing back the interviews whilst reading the transcripts to ensure completeness.

For the interviews with participants the semi structured approach used allowed the researcher to ask open ended questions and helped avoid imposing opinions and assumptions onto the interviewee [25]. Participants had 'free reign' to respond how they wished. To avoid any leading or cohesion, the researcher used brief questions with very little interruption once the participant was responding. Interviews ranged between 45 to 55 min in length, with one participant completing the interview in under 30 min despite the best attempts of the researcher to encourage expansion on the answers provided. Interview sessions were conducted Pre-programme phase 1 (initial 12-week programme). Eight participants were interviewed (Table 1). All participants were approached by Mark Cortnage when attending TAP training sessions and asked if they would like to be interviewed.

Table 1. Participant demographics and phase(s) when interviewed.

Name	Age	BMI (kg/m^2)
Mr C	40	49.9
Mr E	43	39.6
Mr B	50	44.7
Mr R	43	38.9
Mr T	35	32.1
Mr C	51	28.2
Mr F	58	29.1
Mr S	54	32.4

Analysis

Thematic content analysis was used for qualitative analysis of interview data, allowing for a rich, complex account of the interviews to be used to identify themes with detailed meanings [26]. The method provides the means to explore experiences and feelings in separate specific accounts (in relation to questions). As outlined by Braun and Clarke [27], the ability of this method to reflect the reality of experiences shared and to 'unpick the surface of reality' justifies its choice for use here. Responses generated by the semi-structured interviews held at baseline and at the end of the intervention were coded using a thematic approach.

Coding was conducted using Braun and Clarke [27] 'Phases of Analysis', a six stage process that helped the researcher conceptualise the process of thematic analysis) (Table 2). Though recognised more as a guide than a set of rules, the researcher adhered closely to the guidance set out.

Table 2. Phases of analysis used to develop themes.

Phase	Process Description
1	Transcribing of the data. Generation of ideas
2	Generation of codes. Process conducted across the entire data set as opposed to individual interviews.
3	Searching for themes.
4	Reviewing the themes. A review to ensure that the themes align to the codes.
5	Defining and naming of themes.
6	Producing a report based on the themes.

The thematic analysis was conducted manually to enable the researcher to remain close to the data, gaining a thorough understanding of the interviews. Different coloured pens were used to identify and represent themes, providing a visual representation which facilitated a quick glance method of identifying theme development across large swathes of data. On completion of the interviews, the researcher had formed an idea of the types of themes that were present in the data and spent time uncovering as much detail on those as possible when conducting the analysis. Once a theme began to emerge, even vague references such as single words were highlighted, enabling analyses to recognise their contribution to the overall picture.

3. Analysis

The lived experiences of men who participated in the programme are presented through themes identified related to health, football and diet. Four themes were uncovered through thematic content analysis of the interview transcripts, and these are further developed in the discussion (Table 3).

Table 3. TAP pre-programme interview themes.

TAP Programme: Recognised Interview Themes
Attribution of weight gain
Concerns over health and weight
Prior dietary attempts
Feelings about being overweight/obese

This section provides interview findings focusing on the male relationships with food and diet. The men openly discussed the period into which they began to gain weight and suggestions as to the cause, their feelings as to what it is like to be overweight. We can see how perceptions of lifestyle restricts good eating practices and relate to how the men attributed weight gain to two externalised factors; family and employment, providing insight suggesting that they deemed the condition to be out of their control [28]. Analysis outlined strong habitual and routine practices and lack of activity that were viewed by the men as central to weight management. Furthermore, two men had engaged heavily in cyclic dietary behaviours with the period of weight regain significantly shorter than the period of weight loss. Health was seen as of some concern by the men but there was little inclination before joining the programme to address levels of risk. Low self-esteem was prevalent, with negative portrayals of body image manifesting as self-objectification further accompanied by accounts of external sigmatisation.

3.1. Attribution of Weight Gain

It was made evident that lifestyle events decreased the opportunity to exercise. Conversations suggested three reasons for weight gain: lifestyle (including family commitments), occupation supporting a decrease in activity and poor, habitually led food choices. Often, the termination of exercise and the entrance into an alternative, often family centred lifestyle happened simultaneously, and the men would often view them as being incompatible by suggesting that a lifestyle event prevented exercise rather than integrating the two.

> Mr R: ... *I suppose since when the kids arrived. I've always been quite active, always played football, always done something and then the kids came along, that stopped so before you know it you're not younger I was eating the same sort of stuff because you're exercising it's going off ... burning it off, but stopping the exercise. It's because there's less time you're eating more convenient.*

Sobal, Rauschenbach and Frongillo [29] 10-year longitudinal study suggested single men after marriage had a mean weigh gain of 7.4 kg over that period, for men who were already married at baseline, weight increase was 5.8 kg. The 16 year study conducted by Mata et al., [30] suggest significant weight gain in married men of up to up to 0.833 kg/m^2 over that period. Weight increase was determined despite controlling for weight-related behaviours such as age, children, employment suggesting weight gain would be difficult to attribute to a single influence or event rather a whole-lifestyle approach. With around a third of adults spending their life in work, levels of occupational activity can have a significant impact on total daily energy expenditure [31]. The 2016 study by Chin, Nam and Lee [32] posit that managerial occupations, with less activity related tasks were significantly associated with lower aerobic exercise engagement outside of the workplace and suggest how influence on one aspect of lifestyle can impact on another.

> Mr E: *I suppose ... I mean, there's more pressure at work now because I've got more of a high ... more of a managerial role. So, it has ... where work roles changed so there's more responsibility and more time there. So, there's less sort of I suppose flexibility in when you eat and stuff like that but I need something quick and get on with it.*

> Mr C: *I have been putting on weight for years, Mark. I stopped playing football about the age of 35–40ish but because I run my own business, well, I can manage my work when I play football, training and stuff like that, and I wasn't eating as much, but when I stopped playing football and started to settle into life and with having my own business and taking clients out, as you do when you have clients, you take them out for a meal, or a drink and the easier life in relation to social events was like the big thing, so I started to put the weight on.*

A slew of research have suggested that the rise in obesity prevalence coincides increased levels of physical inactivity, wider food choice and unstructured eating behaviours, etc. [33–35]. Recognising strong associations between sedentary behaviour and obesity [36,37], the TAP men provided rare insight into how accessibility to convenience foods coupled with sedentary behaviour contributed to their gradual weight gain.

> Mr R: *Then you probably have a cup of tea with some biscuits although you didn't need it but they're there and you go down that slippery slope and possibly if there was a beer, you'd go and have a beer or something.*

> Mr E: Crisps. *If they're not in the house, it doesn't bother me but if they are in the house, I'll have to have a packet.*

> Mr C: *I think there may be something about starchy stuff that makes you sort of addicted, but I know for a fact that chocolate and crisps are one of my biggest fall-downs. I will be sitting there or might be driving somewhere, and I put a Mars Bar in my mouth rather than an orange or something like that.*

Recognition by participants that they do not need the food suggests that restraint was felt to be beyond them. Despite best intentions, the desire to eat tempting food, whether consciously or not overrides individuals intended behaviours. Regular consumption of treats promotes a relationship between sensory signals and the feeling of satiety that the food presents.

> Mr E: *You know, I've just sat a bit in the evening you know, you're comfortable, you are relaxed, chilled watching the telly or something like that ... my biggest downfall which I'm concentrating on at the moment is I like to pick in the evening. It wouldn't necessarily bother me if I don't eat during the day.*

Mr E provided insight to support research hypothesis that distracted eating has been shown to increase energy consumption [38,39]. The repetitive nature of this eating pattern highlights habitually unconscious consumption practices. One method which has some efficacy in arresting distracted eating is to improve attentiveness when eating and may be a beneficial approach under such circumstances [38,40].

> I: *So, what foods do you know you shouldn't eat but find hard to resist?*
>
> Mr S: *Probably crisps . . . probably savouries more than sweets you know. You know, if somebody said to me in the evening, sitting down do you want a bar of chocolate or a tub of Pringles, I'll go for Pringles.*

This emphasises the potential for convenience to overwrite intentions. Over consumption of regular meals was not a focus of blame, rather confectionary items were. Evening inactivity is unlikely not be the primary reason for daily positive energy, rather a combination of Total Daily Energy Expenditure exceeded through a combination of high fat and high sugar consumption and sedentary behaviours. Research outlines how sedentary aspects can influence poor food choices [41] with suggestions that a combination of reward cues such as stress, boredom and habit are responsible [42,43] and may outline the reasons as to why these men engage in these snacking activities after work.

3.2. Concerns over Health and Weight

The age in which weight gain were thought to have emerged were varied and attributed to external factors and indicated that participants had little motivation to address them once recognised. Three participants mentioned health without the topic being directly addressed and outlined a possible maturing of perceptions in some which contrasts with suggestions that men have little concern for their health or take measures to seek help [44–46]. However, all three respondents had prior health concerns, which positively influenced their perceptions and motivations to address them. Research does suggest that men, post health 'scare' may be more receptive to intervention [47,48]. Mr C worked in IT and largely sedentary throughout the day, participating in little or no exercise at other times. Mr E worked in the Information Technology (IT) field as a manager. His working day was of a sedentary nature and similarly to Mr C, he had developed underlying health conditions in relation to his weight and yet had performed little in the way of preventive action to address these.

> I: *What concerns do you have about being overweight?*
>
> Mr C: *Well, my biggest concern is that after putting on a lot of weight I had a heart attack about 15 years ago, so I don't want to go back into that situation again. I've had no problem since then, but a lot of the problem was due to diabetes. I want to see my days out; I want to be single again and enjoy life instead of carrying on being fat.*
>
> Mr E: *I need to lose weight to help with my blood pressure and get me off the tablets because I hate taking tablets at the best of times and I have to take a stupid amount now. What is it, four tablets I take a day . . . and if I lose weight there's no reason why I then have to take . . . you know, or the doses come down you know?*

Mr B worked in a routine classified occupation as a delivery driver and had had a battery of tests performed a year before joining the programme. Most of his daily routine was driving, taking cargo from one destination to another. He performed very little exercise prior to joining the programme. His cholesterol, blood pressure and resting heart rate were normal (supported through the medication mentioned), and he had lost and regained five and a half stone, and which had culminated into concerns about diabetes due to this rapid weight gain. Despite his health concerns, Mr B. attended intermittently (citing that work commitments prevented his regular attendance).

> Mr B: *Yeah, same with cholesterol as well, that was it, cholesterol test they did. That was right in the middle, that was 5, fine. Before I lost my $5\frac{1}{2}$ stone last year, I put it all back*

on in less than a year ... You could say that my blood sugar level now may be a lot higher because I put it on so quickly, so again. So, I'm aware and conscious that there's health issues, if you know what I mean.

The remaining men only discussed health when the topic was pursued by the researcher and answers focused more on levels of fitness and age rather than the risk of disease associated with being overweight or obese. Other than for two men, preventative approaches to ill-health seemed of little concern, suggesting a disconnect between the benefits of exercise, good diet and reduced health risk. Mr R worked as a car salesman at the time of interview and had a mainly sedentary occupation and though he would take the occasional walk at the weekends, he remained sedentary in his spare time and recognised that his limited fitness motivated him to enroll on the programme. Health was not a motivator for enrolment and only mentioned slight concern of health risk when questioned. Prior to joining the programme he appeared to have done very little to address these concerns.

I: *Which concerns do you have about being overweight such as health for instance?*

Mr R: *Yeah, it is like short of breath probably if you are overweight and if you, do you know even because I don't do any exercise in the winter. So, if you have to find anything out like a couple of months we were in London with my son and we had to go up the escalator in the underground and I was knackered. The same escalator as like eight years ago when I used to work there. I used to fly up and down and now it is like ... that's it. It was absolutely a killer. I was short of breath.*

Mr R: *I suppose I've never really had any health concerns, but I suppose as I'm getting older and you see everybody else that you know ... it's slowly started to drift in the back of your mind your bodies sort of telling you you've got to start doing something.*

Although action was taken by some men to address health concerns, the majority appeared indifferent. Considering their age, reticence may be attributed to embarrassment and/or fear to express themselves [49] or attributed to male gendered performances relating to health risk [50].

3.3. Prior Dietary Attempts

The following section displays attempts by the researcher to uncover efforts by the men to redress increased weight in particularly, their level of engagement with diets and of the level of success. Recognising that TAP was primarily a nutrition programme, with an aim to help men to lose and maintain weight suggested that long term maintenance of weight had not been achieved prior to joining. However, information related to prior dietary attempts would help address the lack of research regarding men and diets.

Mr B: *Huh, I've done all sorts of different sorts of diets, Huh, um last year I did a really good healthy eating, I wouldn't call it diet. But it's smaller amounts of food, more regularly, uh, maintaining your blood sugar level so you don't get cravings, you don't feel hungry and that worked for the time I did it. But then I put all the weight back on after ... Yeah, $5\frac{1}{2}$ stone, uh in 18 weeks.*

I: *Gosh, so you rebounded big time mate.*

Mr B: *Yeah, you know down, personal training, uh badminton lessons 5 times a week and then yeah, just put it all back on. You need to maintain that so you can say eat one day whatever you want and then six days. And then when it's you on your own you go—ah—I'll make it 2 then I'll make it 3 and then it just slips back.*

Mr B: *I did Slimming World probably 6 years ago.*

I: *How did that go?*

Mr B: *Lost 5 stone on that and put all that back on ... there's a 5 stone mark here isn't there, mean mentally when I get to that mark I stop.*

Evidence highlights that men are averse to diets which are embodied as a 'purely female' pursuit [51], with exercise preferred as a means to control weight [52,53]. Men are more inclined to favour individualised, structured and fact-based dietary approaches [54] and once engaged in weight loss, are shown to lose weight more quickly than women [55]. Mr B suggests a rebound will be expected at the 5 stone mark and may hinder further help seeking although with Mr B weight loss achievement was through several days per week of activity and may explain how football is a motivator for participation [56]. Although 18 weeks of activity and weight loss is admirable for Mr B, we are presented with an individual who from a sedentary state, with little exercise conditioning participated in activity daily. Successful weight maintenance strategies outlined by Ramage et al., [57] are associated with decreased energy intake, higher quality food choice, increased activity and behavioural control around food. Recounting two rather successful weight loss attempts followed by weight gain for Mr B suggests that the plethora of facilitators for maintenance had not been accommodated or integrated into lifestyle to such an extent that the behavioural and physical adaptations required to support maintenance become routine. If withdrawal from the sport was forced upon him through, e.g., injury then re-engagement may be difficult unless acclimatisation had been achieved.

With earlier evidence suggesting [6,7] that older men are risk averse and more inclined to see help around health, the dietary patterns of weight loss accompanied by continued high-risk behaviour inducing weight gain, suggest otherwise and highlight a cyclic approach to dieting.

> Mr C.: *So, I started to put the weight on but I sort of 'yo-yo' dieted. I would go on a diet and lose about 3 stones and then I would put it all back on again.*

Rapid and large gains in weight observed in some men over short periods of time reflect high-risk behaviours seen within this group. Rapid regains are associated with reduced resting energy expenditure (REE) [58] and weight cyclers can develop poorer hormonal and metabolic profiles [59]. The participants most affected by persistent weight cycling were unable to show restraint or recognise harm. Although this approach is not solely related to men, evidence does suggest that this is a masculinised health risk behaviour [60,61]. Research on male weight cycling is limited and more commonly addressed in sporting related research [62–64] and yet we can see (above) that for some men losing weight is referred to as an achievement and a natural approach to weight loss rather than maintenance. Investigations in male weight cycling should be considered specifically for men outside of sporting circles and their perception of weight maintenance.

3.4. Feelings about Being Overweight/Obese

It was felt that an exploration of what being overweight or obese felt to the men. We see how the men refer to having excess weight in derogatory terms, such as 'slug', 'crap' portraying self-objectification manifesting as feelings of worthlessness, shame [65] which individually or in combination, support a perpetuation of negative food and activity related behaviours [66,67]. Comments also bring into focus the relationship between weight status and mental health state.

> I: *How does it feel to be overweight?*
>
> Mr E: *I don't like it.*
>
> I: *What sort of feelings does it give you . . . ?*
>
> Mr E: *I feel pretty crap . . . you know, I sort of like get up in the morning and whatever and walked past a mirror and I think, look at that gut . . . but I know I should do something about it. It makes you feel pretty down really to be totally honest.*
>
> Mr T: *It just makes me feel like a slug. It just makes you feel a bit depressed or whatever.*
>
> Mr R: *Sluggish, tired, yeah. Low self-esteem.*

Below, we are further greeted by uncertainty over weight status and brings into clarity a lack of awareness of risk. We are also presented with a lack of knowledge between exercise adaptation, ageing and body size with lower-than-expected performance attributed to weight. A common occurrence with new starters on the programmes was an expectation by participants that they would be able to perform on the pitch to a similar level than before they had retired from playing. This was alleviated through a periodisation approach that supported a gradual increase in intensity over the 12-week period although enthusiasm to perform at a level consistent with their youth was rarely blunted and had to be continuously monitored to reduce injury.

> Mr F: *I don't like it because I've never been overweight . . . . . . but it's more . . . I mean, I'm overweight I wouldn't say . . . I suppose technically I'm obese I would imagine from the way they do it now. . . . but I don't feel huge when I'm walking around all day or anything like that . . . . . . but I notice it when I play five-a-side and my legs get tired like they never did before and I'm sure that must be as much weight as age.*

> Mr E: *Because I don't feel big . . . because of the size of my chest and stuff like that, I sort of hide behind that, well I'm a big lad, you know? Chest, I've got a big chest and I've got some boobs now but . . . I've got a huge chest you know, and I look at it and I just went, oh! When I saw a picture, I went core blimey, you are a big lad but my arms are thin, my legs are thin, I just look like a barrel. Yeah, it's that and I think if I could lose that . . .*

The previous example highlight the potential for mental health to be affected as a result, with feelings of depression openly mentioned and in contrast to the expected stoic response expected [68]. The reciprocal association between obesity and depression has been repeatedly shown [69–71]. Information as to whether obesity causes depression or visa-versa remains uncertain [69] and by asking such a question, this research could have further contributed to that debate.

Improvements in wellbeing for men can be achieved through increases in physical activity, greater peer support and social integration, etc., and presented as a mechanism to alleviate depressive symptoms [72,73]. However, as with most interventions targeting men to date, these are reactive approaches, whereas pro-active intervention, prior to development of symptoms may be a far more effective strategy.

In this study, men reported the absence of health professionals enquiring into how they felt about their obesity. When men are contemplating making lifestyle changes that can positively impact on their weight, the lack of intervention can be considered a missed opportunity. Guidance highlights that physical activity performed regularly can contribute to management of obesity [74]. Healthcare professionals have been identified as being key when promoting health enhancing behaviours such as physical activity [75]. In preparing to intervene, it is also important that healthcare professionals are aware of the behaviours that men demonstrated to deflect their discomfort of being overweight such as being stoic, macho or humorous, as well as the detrimental impact that negative feelings of being obese have on mental wellbeing. Further training and education could be helpful to enhance the preparedness of the Health Care Practitioner to routinely ask men about their feelings about being overweight. This can establish a platform to intervene, especially when men have presented at healthcare settings under their volition.

In alignment with research consensus that for men in particular, recognition of excess body weight risk does not necessarily manifest into a modifying behaviour [76,77] it was recognised that upon recruitment, none of the men in TAP were considered well placed to self-motivate and may have felt vulnerable and open to potential ridicule when joining the programme. Their decision to engage, however, appears to have contributed to levels of confidence and through participation with like-minded individuals in similar circumstances, appears to have helped foster the solidarity that was targeted within the intervention design. Alongside on-programme peer support, peer networks to aid recruitment have been shown as a viable strategy to improve uptake [53].

Stigmatisation is a common accompaniment to being overweight/obese and again associated with negative food related behaviours [78,79]. In addition to self-objectification, perceptions of image extend to other's perception of the subject that even the closest of relationships may be strained by, with a belief that the individual is viewed with disgust. Furthermore, we see (below) how shopping for suitable clothing induces frustration, stress inducing and further perpetuate feelings of shame.

> Mr C: *I have been yo-yoing up and down for years Mark. It's been a problem. I think you get comfortable—my daughter nags me to death, she's healthy and she's quite fit and my partner is too and my kids are all quite slim so I am like the 'blob' of the family and so to a degree it tends to get a bit depressing after a while when you hear that and sometimes when you hear it so often, you think I can't be arsed. But I've got to this stage now where I'm sitting there thinking that I'm going to meetings and I looking at mirrors and I'm wearing a shirt and tie and I'd like to be wearing a suit but I can't get into that suit because I can't get one in my size so I think I'm trying to focus the mind now and trying to get back to a simple way. Ideally, in my case, I'd love to lose 10 stone.*
>
> *Personally, at times I feel depressed, well maybe not depressed. I feel down, what gets to me the worst is buying clothes and you go into a shop and see a really nice suit and you know they won't have it in my size and a size 54 chest you know is getting quite ridiculous. It's got to stop.*
>
> *I do feel embarrassed to be quite honest because the jokes come thick and fast and you laugh with them as part of your make up and you stick by it—it's not killing anybody is it—it hates fat people.*

Mr C provides insight into how approaches to discuss his weight appear infrequent. There is no mention of medical personal enquiring over his feelings, outlining risk or signposting for possible remediation. Furthermore, suggestions portray that he has experienced indirect responses that may attempt to make light of his weight, in this instance alluding to his eligibility for compensation, whether due to comorbidity or mortality is not made clear. Lastly, we are reminded of his discomfort at having to enrol on a programme that addresses men of a certain weight and may further contribute to a reluctance by men to participate. However, programmes, in this instance, conjuring feelings of resignation of weight status and related comorbidities may be the first step in rehabilitation and posit programmes that align behavioural support on developing acceptance of weight status as an alternative approach.

> Mr C: *You are the first person who has ever asked me that. How do you feel? Yes, I feel shit. I would love not to be part of this programme. I mean, this programme is good and I like it because I like playing football.*

3.5. Final Remarks

Low perception of health status risk is recognised in obese adults [80] with underestimation of weight reporting as less binge eating and eating disorder symptomology. Such behaviour, although at first may appear positive, the lack of awareness of true weight status may lead to an exacerbation of risk.

Evidence from interviews and research highlights attribution where treatment response is influenced by individual perceptions of the condition and its causes [81]. For the participants, attributions were more often externalised, placing the cause of their predicament out of their control. This was is in contrast with research, where internalised causes are more typically dominant, e.g., overeating to obesity [81,82]. External, less 'controllable' behaviours are likely to increase despondency and demotivation, presenting as repeated behaviours contributing to the condition [83] for instance, weight cycling behaviours which has been shown to have a significant relationship with all-cause mortality [84].

Patterns of onset weight gain, exercise, self-image and weight loss were contextualised within the lifestyle behaviours of the men were identified. Personal characteristics and experiences shared provided variable levels of emotional insight, highlighting how low self-esteem and lifestyle constraints, e.g., employment accompanied continued high-risk behaviours rather than intervention: facilitating persistent, yet gradual weight gain despite awareness as to how said behaviours negatively influence health. Self-objectification presented a recurring image of poor self-worth and highlighted nuanced self-esteem. Although discourse focused on body image, detrimental comments associating body size and agility (slug) highlighted particularly male gendered connotations with performance on the pitch and highlighted the benefits of providing a programme focusing on ability and skills development to men rather than match-play alone when referencing self-esteem. A similar intervention strategy had been taken with women to some success [85].

Improvements in food knowledge have been shown to improve self-efficacy by enabling the individual to make informed choices [86,87] and social support derived through regular engagement in sport is also proven to be effective in developing self-esteem [53] both of which were utilised with this programme. However, research suggests that participation in exercise for improvements in image may exacerbate feelings of self-objectification, disordered eating and compromised body esteem [88,89] and should be used with caution when used for motivational development. Theories around masculinity however suggest that engagement in exercise for performance and aesthetic improvement is an inducement for male participation [90,91]. The approach used here concentrated on health improvement through a combined diet and fitness approach since although aesthetic improvements and on-pitch performance and physical performance improved as a result, the protocol was designed to ensure these were not overtly addressed to avoid arresting self-esteem development.

Results indicate that men are vulnerable to cyclic dietary behaviours. Eating during comfort breaks were suggested as having strong associations with weight gain and yet despite the awareness of these actions and health risk, attempts to redress were infrequent and lacked commitment.

Two life course events were attributed to their predicament, namely family and employment with discussions telegraphing a sense of resignation and that weight gain was an inevitable consequence of these life choices. Discourse on their weight status were often tinged with despondency and portrayed an erosion of self-esteem, and yet, despite a keen awareness of both their mental state and the inevitable increase in health risk over the life course were their behaviours to continue, action to induce sustainable positive change were not made evident, with attempts to redress being infrequent and non-committal.

The men placed significant emphasis on activity as being a primary regulator of weight and highlighted poor awareness of the multiple negative influences on weight status other than comfort eating. In this regard, and as provided through TAP, men would benefit from incentives that have an educational component that helps develop a holistic understanding of weight and lifestyle that aligns more keenly to their gendered perceptions.

Sharing these findings with services focused on weight loss in men such as commercial and statutory health providers could be helpful in establishing weight loss goals that were not only realistic and sustainable but also seen as credible and as such inclusive of those men who aspired to change their weight loss status and improve their health profiles.

Author Contributions: Conceptualization, M.C.; methodology, M.C.; formal analysis, M.C.; investigation, M.C.; writing—original draft preparation, M.C. and A.P.; writing—Review and Editing M.C. and A.P. All authors have read and agreed to the published version of the manuscript.

Funding: This research received no external funding.

Institutional Review Board Statement: The study was conducted according to the guidelines of the Declaration of Helsinki, and approved by the Faculty (of Medical Science) Research Ethics Panel (FREP) of Anglia Ruskin University (Ref: NS/jc/FMSFREP/15-026 23 June 2015).

Informed Consent Statement: Informed consent was obtained from all subjects involved in the study.

Data Availability Statement: The data presented in this study are available on request from the corresponding author. The data are not publicly available due to ethical restriction.

Acknowledgments: We would like to acknowledge the football coach, Stephen Morgan who provided his time to the programme for free. Thanks go to all the participants of TAP.

Conflicts of Interest: The authors declare no conflict of interest.

References

1. Sabinsky, M.S.; Toft, U.; Raben, A.; Holm, L. Overweight men's motivations and perceived barriers towards weight loss. *Eur. J. Clin. Nutr.* **2007**, *61*, 526–531. [CrossRef]
2. Mahalik, J.; Burns, S.; Syzdek, M. Masculinity and perceived normative health behaviors as predictors of men's health behaviors. *Soc. Sci. Med.* **2007**, *64*, 2201–2209. [CrossRef]
3. Vogel, D.L.; Heimerdinger-Edwards, S.R.; Hammer, J.H.; Hubbard, A. "Boys don't cry": Examination of the links between endorsement of masculine norms, self-stigma, and help-seeking attitudes for men from diverse backgrounds. *J. Couns. Psychol.* **2011**, *58*, 368–382. [CrossRef] [PubMed]
4. Vogel, D.L.; Wade, N.G.; Hackler, A.H. Perceived public stigma and the willingness to seek counseling: The mediating roles of self-stigma and attitudes toward counseling. *J. Couns. Psychol.* **2007**, *54*, 40–50. [CrossRef]
5. Marcos, J.; Avile's, N.; del Rio Lozano, M.; Cuadros, J.; del Mar Garccia Calvente, M. Performing masculinity, influencing health: A qualitative mixed-methods study of young spanish men. *Glob. Health Act.* **2013**, *6*, 21134. [CrossRef]
6. Ebner, N.C.; Freund, A.M.; Baltes, P.B. Developmental changes in personal goal orientation from young to late adulthood: From striving for gains to maintenance and prevention of losses. *Psychol. Aging* **2006**, *21*, 664–678. [CrossRef] [PubMed]
7. Li, L.; Cazzell, M.; Zeng, L.; Liu, H. Are there gender differences in young vs. aging brains under risk decision-making? An optical brain imaging study. *Brain Imaging Behav.* **2017**, *11*, 1085–1098. [CrossRef] [PubMed]
8. Springer, K.W.; Mouzon, D.M.; Journal, S.; Behavior, S.; June, N. "Macho Men" and Preventive Health Care: Implications for Older Men in Different Social Classes. *J. Health Soc. Behav.* **2014**, *52*, 212–227. [CrossRef] [PubMed]
9. National Statistics Health Survey for England 2019: Overweight and Obesity in Adults and Children. 2019. Available online: https://files.digital.nhs.uk/9D/4195D5/HSE19-Overweight-obesity-rep.pdf (accessed on 14 October 2021).
10. National Statistics Changing Trends in Mortality by Leading Causes of Death, England and Wales: 2001 to 2018. 2020. Available online: https://www.ons.gov.uk/peoplepopulationandcommunity/birthsdeathsandmarriages/deaths/articles/changingtrendsinmortalitybyleadingcausesofdeathenglandandwales/2001to2018 (accessed on 13 October 2021).
11. Ogden, J.; Clementi, C. The Experience of Being Obese and the Many Consequences of Stigma. *J. Obes.* **2010**, *2010*, 429098. [CrossRef]
12. Puhl, R.; Brownell, K.D. Ways of coping with obesity stigma: Review and conceptual analysis. *Eat. Behav.* **2003**, *4*, 53–78. [CrossRef]
13. Alegria Drury, C.A.; Louis, M. Exploring the Association Between Body Weight, Stigma of Obesity, and Health Care Avoidance. *J. Am. Acad. Nurse Pract.* **2002**, *14*, 554–561. [CrossRef]
14. Lozano-Sufrategui, L.; Carless, D.; Pringle, A.; Sparkes, A.; McKenna, J. "Sorry Mate, You're Probably a Bit Too Fat to Be Able to Do Any of These": Men's Experiences of Weight Stigma. *Int. J. Mens Health* **2016**, *15*, 4–23. [CrossRef]
15. Naughton, P.; McCarthy, M.; McCarthy, S. Acting to self-regulate unhealthy eating habits. An investigation into the effects of habit, hedonic hunger and self-regulation on sugar consumption from confectionery foods. *Food Qual. Prefer.* **2015**, *46*, 173–183. [CrossRef]
16. Wenger, E. *Communities of Practice: Learning, Meaning, and Identity*; Cambridge University Press: Cambridge, UK, 1998.
17. Lefkowich, M.; Richardson, N.; Robertson, S. "If We Want to Get Men in, Then We Need to Ask Men What They Want": Pathways to Effective Health Programing for Men. *Am. J. Mens Health* **2017**, *11*, 1512–1524. [CrossRef]
18. Bass, B.M.; Riggio, R.E. *Transformational Leadership*, 2nd ed.; Erlbaum Associates: Mahwah, NJ, USA, 2006.
19. Ahern, A.L.; Olson, A.D.; Aston, L.M.; Jebb, S.A. Weight Watchers on prescription: An observational study of weight change among adults referred to Weight Watchers by the NHS. *BMC Public Health* **2011**, *11*, 434. [CrossRef] [PubMed]
20. Stubbs, R.J.; Pallister, C.; Whybrow, S.; Avery, A.; Lavin, J. Weight Outcomes Audit for 34,271 Adults Referred to a Primary Care/Commercial Weight Management Partnership Scheme. *Obes. Facts* **2011**, *4*, 113–120. [CrossRef] [PubMed]
21. Mauro Manzoni, G. Internet-Based Behavioral Interventions for Obesity: An Updated Systematic Review. *Clin. Pract. Epidemiol. Ment. Health* **2011**, *7*, 19–28. [CrossRef]
22. Economic and Social Research Council ESRC Framework for Research Ethics (FRE) 2010 Updated September 2012. 2012. Available online: https://esrc.ukri.org/ (accessed on 24 June 2015).
23. ten Have, M.; van der Heide, A.; Mackenbach, J.P.; de Beaufort, I.D. An ethical framework for the prevention of overweight and obesity: A tool for thinking through a programme's ethical aspects. *Eur. J. Public Health* **2013**, *23*, 299–305. [CrossRef]
24. Etikan, I. Comparison of Convenience Sampling and Purposive Sampling. *Am. J. Theor. Appl. Stat.* **2016**, *5*, 1–4. [CrossRef]
25. Britten, N. Qualitative Research: Qualitative interviews in medical research. *BMJ* **1995**, *311*, 251–253. [CrossRef]
26. Vaismoradi, M.; Turunen, H.; Bondas, T. Content analysis and thematic analysis: Implications for conducting a qualitative descriptive study: Qualitative descriptive study. *Nurs. Health Sci.* **2013**, *15*, 398–405. [CrossRef]
27. Braun, V.; Clarke, V. Using thematic analysis in psychology. *Qual. Res. Psychol.* **2006**, *3*, 77–101. [CrossRef]

28. Deci, E.L.; Ryan, R.M. Self-determination theory: A macrotheory of human motivation, development, and health. *Can. Psychol. Can.* **2008**, *49*, 182–185. [CrossRef]
29. Bove, C.F.; Sobal, J.; Rauschenbach, B.S. Food choices among newly married couples: Convergence, conflict, individualism, and projects. *Appetite* **2003**, *40*, 25–41. [CrossRef]
30. Mata, J.; Richter, D.; Schneider, T.; Hertwig, R. How cohabitation, marriage, separation, and divorce influence BMI: A prospective panel study. *Health Psychol.* **2018**, *37*, 948–958. [CrossRef] [PubMed]
31. Allman-Farinelli, M.A.; Chey, T.; Merom, D.; Bauman, A.E. Occupational risk of overweight and obesity: An analysis of the Australian Health Survey. *J. Occup. Med. Toxicol.* **2010**, *5*, 14. [CrossRef] [PubMed]
32. Chin, D.L.; Nam, S.; Lee, S.-J. Occupational factors associated with obesity and leisure-time physical activity among nurses: A cross sectional study. *Int. J. Nurs. Stud.* **2016**, *57*, 60–69. [CrossRef] [PubMed]
33. Bellisle, F. Meals and snacking, diet quality and energy balance. *Physiol. Behav.* **2014**, *134*, 38–43. [CrossRef] [PubMed]
34. Roman, G. Eating Patterns, Physical Activity and Their Association with Demographic Factors in the Population Included in the Obesity Study in Romania (ORO Study). *Acta Endocrinol. Buchar.* **2016**, *12*, 47–51. [CrossRef]
35. Eknoyan, G. A History of Obesity, or How What Was Good Became Ugly and Then Bad. *Adv. Chronic Kidney Dis.* **2006**, *13*, 421–427. [CrossRef]
36. Rogerson, M.C.; Le Grande, M.R.; Dunstan, D.W.; Magliano, D.J.; Murphy, B.M.; Salmon, J.; Gardiner, P.A.; Jackson, A.C. Television Viewing Time and 13-year Mortality in Adults with Cardiovascular Disease: Data from the Australian Diabetes, Obesity and Lifestyle Study (AusDiab). *Heart Lung Circ.* **2016**, *25*, 829–836. [CrossRef] [PubMed]
37. Raynor, H.A.; Looney, S.M.; Steeves, E.A.; Spence, M.; Gorin, A.A. The Effects of an Energy Density Prescription on Diet Quality and Weight Loss: A Pilot Randomized Controlled Trial. *J. Acad. Nutr. Diet.* **2012**, *112*, 1397–1402. [CrossRef] [PubMed]
38. Robinson, E.; Aveyard, P.; Daley, A.; Jolly, K.; Lewis, A.; Lycett, D.; Higgs, S. Eating attentively: A systematic review and meta-analysis of the effect of food intake memory and awareness on eating. *Am. J. Clin. Nutr.* **2013**, *97*, 728–742. [CrossRef] [PubMed]
39. Spence, M.; Livingstone, M.B.E.; Hollywood, L.E.; Gibney, E.R.; O'Brien, S.A.; Pourshahidi, L.K.; Dean, M. A qualitative study of psychological, social and behavioral barriers to appropriate food portion size control. *Int. J. Behav. Nutr. Phys. Act.* **2013**, *10*, 92. [CrossRef] [PubMed]
40. Arch, J.J.; Brown, K.W.; Goodman, R.J.; Della Porta, M.D.; Kiken, L.G.; Tillman, S. Enjoying food without caloric cost: The impact of brief mindfulness on laboratory eating outcomes. *Behav. Res. Ther.* **2016**, *79*, 23–34. [CrossRef]
41. Griffith, D.M.; Wooley, A.M.; Allen, J.O. "I'm Ready to Eat and Grab Whatever I Can Get": Determinants and Patterns of African American Men's Eating Practices. *Health Promot. Pract.* **2013**, *14*, 181–188. [CrossRef]
42. Pool, E.; Delplanque, S.; Coppin, G.; Sander, D. Is comfort food really comforting? Mechanisms underlying stress-induced eating. *Food Res. Int.* **2015**, *76*, 207–215. [CrossRef]
43. Koball, A.M.; Meers, M.R.; Storfer-Isser, A.; Domoff, S.E.; Musher-Eizenman, D.R. Eating when bored: Revision of the Emotional Eating Scale with a focus on boredom. *Health Psychol.* **2012**, *31*, 521–524. [CrossRef]
44. Yousaf, O.; Grunfeld, E.A.; Hunter, M.S. A systematic review of the factors associated with delays in medical and psychological help-seeking among men. *Health Psychol. Rev.* **2015**, *9*, 264–276. [CrossRef] [PubMed]
45. Galdas, P.M.; Cheater, F.; Marshall, P. Men and health help-seeking behaviour: Literature review. *J. Adv. Nurs.* **2005**, *49*, 616–623. [CrossRef]
46. Seidler, Z.E.; Dawes, A.J.; Rice, S.M.; Oliffe, J.L.; Dhillon, H.M. The role of masculinity in men's help-seeking for depression: A systematic review. *Clin. Psychol. Rev.* **2016**, *49*, 106–118. [CrossRef]
47. Horwood, J.P.; Avery, K.N.; Metcalfe, C.; Donovan, J.L.; Hamdy, F.C.; Neal, D.E.; Lane, J.A. Men's knowledge and attitudes towards dietary prevention of a prostate cancer diagnosis: A qualitative study. *BMC Cancer* **2014**, *14*, 812. [CrossRef]
48. Mróz, L.W.; Chapman, G.E.; Oliffe, J.L.; Bottorff, J.L. Men, Food, and Prostate Cancer: Gender Influences on Men's Diets. *Am. J. Mens Health* **2011**, *5*, 177–187. [CrossRef]
49. Fish, J.A.; Prichard, I.; Ettridge, K.; Grunfeld, E.A.; Wilson, C. Psychosocial factors that influence men's help-seeking for cancer symptoms: A systematic synthesis of mixed methods research: Psychosocial factors that influence men's help-seeking. *Psychooncology* **2015**, *24*, 1222–1232. [CrossRef] [PubMed]
50. Courtenay, W.H. Constructions of masculinity and their influence on men's well-being: A theory of gender and health. *Soc. Sci.* **2000**, *50*, 1385–1401. [CrossRef]
51. Gough, B. 'Real men don't diet': An analysis of contemporary newspaper representations of men, food and health. *Soc. Sci. Med.* **2007**, *64*, 326–337. [CrossRef] [PubMed]
52. Kiefer, I.; Rathmanner, T.; Kunze, M. Eating and dieting differences in men and women. *J. Mens Health Gend.* **2005**, *2*, 194–201. [CrossRef]
53. Pringle, A.; Zwolinsky, S.; McKenna, J.; Robertson, S.; Daly-Smith, A.; White, A. Health improvement for men and hard-to-engage-men delivered in English Premier League football clubs. *Health Educ. Res.* **2014**, *29*, 503–520. [CrossRef]
54. Robertson, C.; Hoddinott, P.; Stewart, F.; Street, T. Systematic reviews of and integrated report on the quantitative, qualitative and economic evidence base for the management of obesity in men. *Health Technol. Assess.* **2014**, *8*, 1–424. [CrossRef] [PubMed]
55. Pagoto, S.L.; Schneider, K.L.; Oleski, J.L.; Luciani, J.M.; Bodenlos, J.S.; Whited, M.C. Male Inclusion in Randomized Controlled Trials of Lifestyle Weight Loss Interventions. *Obesity* **2012**, *20*, 1234–1239. [CrossRef]

56. Gray, C.M.; Hunt, K.; Mutrie, N.; Anderson, A.S.; Leishman, J.; Dalgarno, L.; Wyke, S. Football Fans in Training: The development and optimization of an intervention delivered through professional sports clubs to help men lose weight, become more active and adopt healthier eating habits. *BMC Public Health* **2013**, *13*, 232. [CrossRef]
57. Ramage, S.; Farmer, A.; Apps Eccles, K.; McCargar, L. Healthy strategies for successful weight loss and weight maintenance: A systematic review. *Appl. Physiol. Nutr. Metab.* **2014**, *39*, 1–20. [CrossRef] [PubMed]
58. Johannsen, D.L.; Knuth, N.D.; Huizenga, R.; Rood, J.C.; Ravussin, E.; Hall, K.D. Metabolic Slowing with Massive Weight Loss despite Preservation of Fat-Free Mass. *J. Clin. Endocrinol. Metab.* **2012**, *97*, 2489–2496. [CrossRef]
59. Mason, C.; Foster-Schubert, K.E.; Imayama, I.; Xiao, L.; Kong, A.; Campbell, K.L.; Duggan, C.R.; Wang, C.-Y.; Alfano, C.M.; Ulrich, C.M.; et al. History of weight cycling does not impede future weight loss or metabolic improvements in postmenopausal women. *Metabolism* **2013**, *62*, 127–136. [CrossRef]
60. Vandello, J.A.; Bosson, J.K. Hard won and easily lost: A review and synthesis of theory and research on precarious manhood. *Psychol. Men Masc.* **2013**, *14*, 101–113. [CrossRef]
61. Gough, B. The psychology of men's health: Maximizing masculine capital. *Health Psychol.* **2013**, *32*, 1–4. [CrossRef]
62. Fortes, L.S.; Costa, B.D.V.; Paes, P.P.; Cyrino, E.S.; Vianna, J.M.; Franchini, E. Effect of rapid weight loss on physical performance in judo athletes: Is rapid weight loss a help for judokas with weight problems? *Int. J. Perform. Anal. Sport* **2017**, *17*, 763–773. [CrossRef]
63. Berkovich, B.-E.; Eliakim, A.; Nemet, D.; Stark, A.H.; Sinai, T. Rapid Weight Loss Among Adolescents Participating In Competitive Judo. *Int. J. Sport Nutr. Exerc. Metab.* **2016**, *26*, 276–284. [CrossRef] [PubMed]
64. Dulloo, A.G.; Montani, J.-P. Pathways from dieting to weight regain, to obesity and to the metabolic syndrome: An overview: Dieting and cardiometabolic risks. *Obes. Rev.* **2015**, *16*, 1–6. [CrossRef] [PubMed]
65. Conradt, M.; Dierk, J.-M.; Schlumberger, P.; Rauh, E.; Hebebrand, J.; Rief, W. Who copes well? Obesity-related coping and its associations with shame, guilt, and weight loss. *J. Clin. Psychol.* **2008**, *64*, 1129–1144. [CrossRef]
66. Hemmingsson, E. A new model of the role of psychological and emotional distress in promoting obesity: Conceptual review with implications for treatment and prevention: Psychoemotional distress in weight gain. *Obes. Rev.* **2014**, *15*, 769–779. [CrossRef] [PubMed]
67. Davenport, K.; Houston, J.E.; Griffiths, M.D. Excessive Eating and Compulsive Buying Behaviours in Women: An Empirical Pilot Study Examining Reward Sensitivity, Anxiety, Impulsivity, Self-Esteem and Social Desirability. *Int. J. Ment. Health Addict.* **2012**, *10*, 474–489. [CrossRef]
68. Schrock, D.; Schwalbe, M. Men, Masculinity, and Manhood Acts. *Annu. Rev. Sociol.* **2009**, *35*, 277–295. [CrossRef]
69. Milaneschi, Y.; Simmons, W.K.; van Rossum, E.F.C.; Penninx, B.W. Depression and obesity: Evidence of shared biological mechanisms. *Mol. Psychiatry* **2019**, *24*, 18–33. [CrossRef] [PubMed]
70. Faith, M.S.; Matz, P.E.; Jorge, M.A. Obesity–depression associations in the population. *J. Psychosom. Res.* **2002**, *53*, 935–942. [CrossRef]
71. Luppino, F.S.; de Wit, L.M.; Bouvy, P.F.; Stijnen, T.; Cuijpers, P.; Penninx, B.W.J.H.; Zitman, F.G. Overweight, Obesity, and Depression: A Systematic Review and Meta-analysis of Longitudinal Studies. *Arch. Gen. Psychiatry* **2010**, *67*, 220. [CrossRef] [PubMed]
72. Drew, R.J.; Morgan, P.J.; Young, M.D. Mechanisms of an eHealth program targeting depression in men with overweight or obesity: A randomised trial. *J. Affect. Disord.* **2022**, *299*, 309–317. [CrossRef] [PubMed]
73. Currier, D.; Lindner, R.; Spittal, M.J.; Cvetkovski, S.; Pirkis, J.; English, D.R. Physical activity and depression in men: Increased activity duration and intensity associated with lower likelihood of current depression. *J. Affect. Disord.* **2020**, *260*, 426–431. [CrossRef] [PubMed]
74. Department of Health and Social Care. 'UK Chief Medical Officers' Physical Activity Guidelines'. September 2019. Available online: https://www.gov.uk/government/publications/physical-activity-guidelines-uk-chief-medical-officers-report (accessed on 24 June 2015).
75. Mutrie, N.; Richards, K.; Lawrie, S.; Mead, G. Can physical activity prevent or treat clinical depression? In *The Exercise Effect on Mental Health: Neurobiological Mechanisms*, 1st ed.; Budde, H., Wegner, M., Budde, H., Wegner, M., Eds.; Routledge: London, UK; CRC Press: New York, NY, USA, 2018; pp. 380–407.
76. Coulson, F.; Ypinazar, V.; Margolis, S. Awareness of risks of overweight among rural Australians. *Rural Remote Health* **2006**. [CrossRef]
77. Avis, N.E.; McKinlay, J.B.; Smith, K.W. Is cardiovascular risk factor knowledge sufficient to influence behavior? *Am. J. Prev. Med.* **1990**, *6*, 137–144. [CrossRef]
78. Sattler, K.M.; Deane, F.P.; Tapsell, L.; Kelly, P.J. Gender differences in the relationship of weight-based stigmatisation with motivation to exercise and physical activity in overweight individuals. *Health Psychol. Open* **2018**, *5*, 2055102918759691. [CrossRef]
79. Schvey, N.A.; Puhl, R.M.; Brownell, K.D. The Impact of Weight Stigma on Caloric Consumption. *Obesity* **2011**, *19*, 1957–1962. [CrossRef] [PubMed]
80. Jones, M.; Grilo, C.M.; Masheb, R.M.; White, M.A. Psychological and behavioral correlates of excess weight: Misperception of obese status among persons with Class II obesity. *Int. J. Eat. Disord.* **2010**, *43*, 628–632. [CrossRef] [PubMed]
81. Brogan, A.; Hevey, D. The structure of the causal attribution belief network of patients with obesity. *Br. J. Health Psychol.* **2009**, *14*, 35–48. [CrossRef] [PubMed]

82. Weiner, B.; Perry, R.P.; Magnusson, J. An attributional analysis of reactions to stigmas. *J. Pers. Soc. Psychol.* **1988**, *55*, 738–748. [CrossRef] [PubMed]
83. Wamsteker, E.W.; Geenen, R.; Zelissen, P.M.J.; van Furth, E.F.; Iestra, J. Unrealistic Weight-Loss Goals among Obese Patients Are Associated with Age and Causal Attributions. *J. Am. Diet. Assoc.* **2009**, *109*, 1903–1908. [CrossRef] [PubMed]
84. Rzehak, P.; Meisinger, C.; Woelke, G.; Brasche, S.; Strube, G.; Heinrich, J. Weight change, weight cycling and mortality in the ERFORT Male Cohort Study. *Eur. J. Epidemiol.* **2007**, *22*, 665–673. [CrossRef] [PubMed]
85. Alleva, J.M.; Martijn, C.; Van Breukelen, G.J.P.; Jansen, A.; Karos, K. Expand Your Horizon: A programme that improves body image and reduces self-objectification by training women to focus on body functionality. *Body Image* **2015**, *15*, 81–89. [CrossRef] [PubMed]
86. Gittelsohn, J.; Anliker, J.A.; Sharma, S.; Vastine, A.E.; Caballero, B.; Ethelbah, B. Psychosocial Determinants of Food Purchasing and Preparation in American Indian Households. *J. Nutr. Educ. Behav.* **2006**, *38*, 163–168. [CrossRef] [PubMed]
87. Beydoun, M.A.; Wang, Y. Do nutrition knowledge and beliefs modify the association of socio-economic factors and diet quality among US adults? *Prev. Med.* **2008**, *46*, 145–153. [CrossRef]
88. Strelan, P.; Hargreaves, D. Reasons for Exercise and Body Esteem: Men's Responses to Self-Objectification. *Sex Roles* **2005**, *53*, 495–503. [CrossRef]
89. Prichard, I.; Tiggemann, M. Relations among exercise type, self-objectification, and body image in the fitness centre environment: The role of reasons for exercise. *Psychol. Sport Exerc.* **2008**, *9*, 855–866. [CrossRef]
90. Gough, B.; Conner, M.T. Barriers to healthy eating amongst men: A qualitative analysis. *Soc. Sci. Med.* **2006**, *62*, 387–395. [CrossRef] [PubMed]
91. De Visser, R.O.; McDonnell, E.J. "Man points": Masculine capital and young men's health. *Health Psychol.* **2013**, *32*, 5–14. [CrossRef] [PubMed]

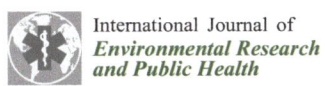

Article

An Exploration of People Living with Parkinson's Experience of Cardio-Drumming; Parkinson's Beats: A Qualitative Phenomenological Study

J. Yoon Irons [1,*], Alison Williams [2], Jo Holland [2] and Julie Jones [3]

1. School of Psychology, College of Health, Psychology and Social Care, University of Derby, Derby DE22 1GB, UK
2. Parkinson's Scotland Office, 1/14 King James VI Business Centre, Friarton Road, Perth PH2 8DY, UK; alison@edinburghparkinsons.org (A.W.); jhollandparkinsons@gmail.com (J.H.)
3. School of Health Sciences, Robert Gordon University, Garthdee Road, Aberdeen AB10 7QG, UK; j.c.jones@rgu.ac.uk
* Correspondence: y.irons@derby.ac.uk

Abstract: Research has shown that physical activity has a range of benefits for people living with Parkinson's (PLwP), improving muscle strength, balance, flexibility, and walking, as well as non-motor symptoms such as mood. Parkinson's Beats is a form of cardio-drumming, specifically adapted for PLwP, and requires no previous experience nor skills. Nineteen PLwP (aged between 55 and 80) took part in the regular Parkinson's Beats sessions in-person or online. Focus group discussions took place after twelve weeks to understand the impacts of Parkinson's Beats. Through the framework analysis, six themes and fifteen subthemes were generated. Participants reported a range of benefits of cardio-drumming, including improved fitness and movement, positive mood, the flow experience, and enhanced social wellbeing. A few barriers to participation were also reported. Future research is justified, and best practice guidelines are needed to inform healthcare professionals, PLwP and their care givers.

Keywords: Parkinson's disease; drumming exercises; flow experience; empowerment; physical activity; mental health; eye-hand coordination; multi-disciplinary; music; healthy ageing

1. Introduction

Parkinson's is the fastest-growing neurodegenerative condition [1]. Ten million people live with Parkinson's worldwide [2], and over 145,000 people in the UK are diagnosed with Parkinson's [3]. Due to the ageing population, the incidence of Parkinson's is expected to continue to rise [4], highlighting the need for effective healthcare interventions to support a growing global community.

There is no cure for Parkinson's, and its exact cause remains unknown. However, increased age, lifestyle, and a complex interaction of environmental and genetic factors are commonly implicated [5]. Parkinson's is characterised by the loss of dopaminergic neurones within the Substantia Nigra Pars Compacta. The progressive loss of neurones results in a decrease in activity of the Nigrostriatal circuits, which increasingly inhibits the Basal Ganglia. Ultimately, this leads to a decrease in or poverty of movement, which is synonymous with Parkinson's. The exact mechanism precipitating neuronal loss in Parkinson's is unknown. Due to the progressive loss of neurones, Parkinson's is now recognised as a broad multi-system condition encompassing over 40 motor and non-motor symptoms [6]. Historically, Parkinson's was regarded solely as a movement disorder [7]; however, non-motor symptoms are now widely recognised as integral to Parkinson's, with apathy, depression, and anxiety being prevalent among the Parkinson's community [4].

The management of Parkinson's is complex, owing to its progressive nature, patient heterogeneity, and symptom diversity. Management is reliant upon medication, which targets dopamine imbalance through a variety of different mechanisms [8]. Moreover, medication efficacy is time limited, with Parkinson's progression necessitating different combinations of medications, taken at increasing dosages, due to the medication's effect wearing off. Thus, with a growing Parkinson's population, and finite benefits from medication, there is a pressing need to develop effective long-term health interventions.

Physical activity (PA) has been hailed as "the new medicine" for Parkinson's; PA is no longer viewed as a complementary intervention, but of equal importance to medication [9]. The interest in PA has been fuelled by the association between PA and the reduced risk of developing Parkinson's [10] and the potential to attenuate symptom progression [11,12]. Systematic reviews highlight that PA results in improved strength, balance, gait, and physical capacity [13–16], as well as improved motor and non-motor symptoms [17–22]. Current guidelines advocate that weekly PA programmes should be prescribed in a progressive manner, including strength, balance, aerobic, gait, and task-specific training focusing on the upper and lower limbs and spine, with emphasis placed on functional movement patterns and large amplitude movements [23]. In addition, the high incidence of apathy in Parkinson's means that to maintain motivation, PA needs to be enjoyable.

Parkinson's Beats

Cardio-drumming programmes or drumming exercises have recently been gaining popularity. Drumming is a relatively high-intensity aerobic exercise involving whole-body movements [24]. A workout ball in a bucket (e.g., [25]), or African drums (e.g., [26]) can be used, as they are easily available and do not require previous training or specific knowledge and skills to play. Drumming exercises combining movement with rhythmic, up-beat music, build enjoyment and support the incremental pace, aiming to increase cardiovascular benefits.

The core of drumming relies on our intrinsic ability, known as entrainment, to tap/play along with the rhythms of music (i.e., synchronising our movement with music/beats). This entrainment is of particular importance for people living with Parkinson's (PLwP), as the music's beats can effectively support the brain to coordinate movements [27,28]. For example, a systematic review of meta-analyses of clinical studies involving music for movement rehabilitation in Parkinson's demonstrated that when music was added to gait training, it resulted in significant improvements of balance, stride length, and walking (measured using the Timed Up and Go test) in PLwP [29]. This is because rhythmic stimulation offers beneficial time-based cues for the brain to plan and be ready to execute the next movement [27]. Applying rhythmic entrainment to drumming exercises, which involve synchronised movements stimulated by beats, Parkinson's Beats is specifically adapted for PLwP to promote large amplitude arm movements, balance through differing drumming techniques, and strength training in the legs. Further, a randomised controlled study highlighted that group-based drumming programmes decreased participants' depression and anxiety, and increased wellbeing and social resilience [30]. Moreover, positive experiences including enjoyment, a sense of control, accomplishments, and social connectedness were reported in a study with mental health service users [31]. To utilise these numerous advantages of drumming, a pilot study was conducted involving eighteen PLwP, where only eight participants took part in drumming and ten participants were in the control group [32]. Following the twice-weekly 6-week West African drum circle intervention, participants in the drumming group demonstrated a statistically significant improvement in the quality-of-life measure (PDQ-39), but no improvements in depression and motor function assessments. In this study, the qualitative assessment was limited to several quotes from participants' diary entries, and no formal qualitative analysis was involved. Therefore, the current study aimed to explore the impacts of a cardio-drumming programme, Parkinson's Beats, which uses a workout ball in a bucket with two sticks. Given the fact that this was only a recently adopted exercise programme for PLwP, the focus of this study was to gain a better understanding of the lived experience of PLwP taking part in Parkinson's Beats using a descriptive phenomenological method [33].

2. Methods

2.1. Design

A qualitative phenomenological research design [34] was used to gain an understanding of the impact of Parkinson's Beats (PB). Adopting a phenomenological approach allows for a greater understanding of and insight into the experience of PLwP who participated in Parkinson's Beats. The descriptive phenomenological approach seeks to explain the nature of things through the way people experience them [34]. Such an approach allows us to capture and describe essential aspects of the participants' experience, to understand their experience in their context, i.e., living with Parkinson's [33]. This study was ethically approved by the Robert Gordon University School of Health Sciences Research Ethics Committee (SREC SHS/22/32).

2.2. Participants

This study adopted a convenience approach to sampling, inviting PLwP who had attended four or more Parkinson's Beats sessions, delivered either online or face-to-face, to participate in a focus group to explore their experiences of participation in Parkinson's Beats. As Parkinson's Beats is an inclusive form of activity and can be adapted to suit all abilities, no restriction was based on stage of Parkinson's, time since diagnosis, or Parkinson's medication. Parkinson's Beats attendees received a participation information sheet via email and provided statements of informed consent prior to participating in the study. Although we did not formally assess eligible participants on their cognitive function, all our participants did not have any form of dementia. They provided statements of informed consent, followed all instructions during the weekly cardio-drumming sessions, and were able to share their thoughts and experiences of Parkinson's Beats at the focus group discussions.

2.3. Data Collection

The qualitative data were gathered through audio-recorded conversations of three focus groups: one in-person group ($n = 9$) and two online groups via Microsoft Teams ($n = 5$ in each group). Focus groups 1 and 2 were conducted immediately following the drumming session; the third was held on a day where there was no drumming.

Focus group discussions were guided by a standardised topic guide incorporating four key areas of interest: (i) their initial thoughts of Parkinson's Beats, (ii) their experience of Parkinson's Beats, (iii) the perceived impact of Parkinson's Beats, and (iv) barriers and motivators to participation in Parkinson's Beats.

All focus groups were facilitated by the same researcher (AW). An additional member of the research team (JH) served as an observer and took field notes to complement the qualitative analysis. All focus groups were recorded, and accurately transcribed.

2.4. Data Analysis

Interview transcripts were analysed following Ritchie and Lewis' framework analysis approach [35], which is commonly used within health-related research [36], and is ideally suited to exploring participants' perceptions, experiences, and values, aligning with the objectives of this research. The framework analysis approach was selected as it offers a flexible approach to identify and describe the data and categorise key patterns to generate themes related to the phenomenon of interest [34]. Using this inductive approach meant that participants' views and opinions dictated the emergence of themes and subthemes. The researchers (AW and JH) grouped themes and subthemes, discussing their scope and nature with the rest of the research team (JJ and JYI), and making any necessary amendments.

3. Results

In total, seven men and twelve women, ranging in age between 55 and 80 years old, took part in the Parkinson's Beats study. Participants ($n = 5$) were excluded from the analysis only if they had attended fewer than four sessions of Parkinson's Beats.

The framework analysis resulted in the identification of six themes and fifteen subthemes. Themes centred upon physical improvements, benefits on mood, cognitive function, social wellbeing, additional benefits, and barriers to participation, as illustrated in Table 1.

Table 1. Themes and subthemes of participants experiences.

Themes	Subthemes with Representative Quotes
1. Physical impact The focus groups were intentionally run following a PB session, to capture participants' immediate respones.	1.1 Immediate post-class physical impact "I am just buzzing after attending the class, like I am ready to take on anything" "I feel energised, and it lasts the rest of the day" 1.2 Functional benefits "Yes, I'm like that—I can reach cupboard shelves that I couldn't reach before" "When I first started doing this—I have a lot of pain with my PD [Parkinson's disease], I have arthritis and I have a lot of issues. I struggle to get up and down the stairs. So I used to get the lift up to my class and the lift down. So about the fourth session I came out of the class and I was chatting away to people and I was at the bottom of the stairs before I realised I had walked down the stairs and I hadn't felt any pain. And it's just the exhilaration of the drumming that had done that" 1.3 Lasting effects "I am not sure if it is because of the drumming, but I have notice my hand writing has improved recently, and my medication has not changed" "On drumming days I'm a lot more [chilled] because I don't have the pain and the stiffness" "I would say the simple action of using your arms and your hand/eye coordination. It really lifts you body and mind"
2. Emotional impact Parkinson's Beats was unanimously perceived to have a positive impact on non-motor symptoms.	2.1 Impact during and immediately after class "Upbeat—you do feel good. You feel up rather than down". Attending Parkinson's Beats also served as a distraction for many, allowing them to forget about their Parkinson's for a period of time: "Actually doing it, I forget about the Parkinson's"; and "I forget about Parkinson's for the rest of that day". "It's amazingly relaxing, the whole thing; and you're concentrating on something other than your tremor. You're concentrating on the drumming and forget about your tremor" 2.2 Distraction and reduced stress "I just love it—it's a selfish thing for me, I love to see people enjoying themselves—it gives so much back to me" "This is fun—if you can find something you can enjoy then you're more likely to keep it up. She [the instructor] makes it fun, she really does" 2.3 Enhanced emotional wellbeing and empowerment "Just enjoy what you can do. Every day is different. Some days you can't do a lot" "You don't have to—that's the beauty of drumming, you are a free spirit, you do what you like. The more you do it, the better you get as well".
3. Impact on cognitive function Participating in Parkinson's Beats presented a cognitive challenge for participants. Participants reported that they enjoyed the challenge of the complex tracks and rhythms.	3.1 Mastering challenges "I like the more complex [music] tracks" "There's more for you to do, it's more enter-taining, you feel more positive at the end of it" "You're pushing yourself more as well because some of the more complex movements at more difficult to achieve" "You have to concentrate so much, and quite a lot of effort put into it". 3.2 Frustrations "That's really important that people don't feel that they have to achieve a standard. Cos there is no standard" "It just makes me so cross that I can't do it as well as I would like to"

Table 1. Cont.

Themes	Subthemes with Representative Quotes
4. Social Benefits The participants had positive experiences of being in a group, enjoyment of making music together, and working with others in a group.	4.1 Working with others "Trying to finish at the same time as everyone else" "Being in tune with others is a great feeling" Participants were clear that "Doing it [drumming] on your own wouldn't be the same"
5. Additional benefits Three subthemes emerged in this theme: music, dance, and the loss of self-consciousness.	5.1 Music "There's something about creating music, dancing to the beat, or drumming to the beat" "It's funny—I do listen to music in a different way now. I'm thinking: How would I move/beat to that music? you know, when you're in the car, and you bang the steering wheel ..." 5.2 Dance "It's more like dancing for me—there's movement in it, and I tend to try to make it into a dance anyway" 5.3 Losing self-consciousness "I like the zoom. I'm not so sure I'd do it if it wasn't on zoom. I'd be so self-conscious, that I was not hitting the drum at the same time that it would put me off" "I like being able to lose all of my frustrations" "Just start making your own noise. Fun. Lash out"
6. Barriers Three potential barriers emerged in the focus group discussions: self-consciousness, retrospection, and the music chosen.	6.1 Self-consciousness "I can't forget about my illness when I'm drumming, because it just make me so cross that I can't do it as well as I would like to. [Told, there's no pressure, the participant responded] the pressure is all at my end". 6.2 Drumming noise "I have a problem—we now have a rabbit living in the house so now I have to quieten down a bit—the rabbit doesn't like it" 6.3 Music choice "A couple of people came once but didn't like the music. Said if it was classical, they would be more likely to join"

3.1. Theme 1. Physical Impact

The focus groups were intentionally run following a Parkinson's Beats session, to capture participants' immediate responses. Experiences of Parkinson's Beats varied from some participants feeling euphoric and energised; further, some participants perceived that they had a good work out.

"I am just buzzing after attending the class, like I am ready to take on anything"

"I feel energised, and it lasts the rest of the day"

"Done some exercise, love the music, love instructor. It's a happy class. You feel you've achieved something as well"

Some participants reported "muscle tiredness" and "some muscle ache" but this was not expressed negatively; rather, these comments attested to the fact that they had a good workout. However, one participant reported that they could no longer do both Parkinson's Beats and Tango class in the same day again, suggesting that Parkinson's Beats was a high-intensity exercise.

In addition to physical benefits, participants also reported functional benefits. These included, but were not limited to, an improved ability to raise their arms with greater ease, so that they were now able to reach top shelves. Improvements to upper limbs were also evidenced by participants reporting a greater ability to use their arms to get out of bed more easily, and increased mobility. In addition, participants also reported perceived reductions in pain, stiffness, and tremors on drumming class days.

"Yes, I'm like that—I can reach cupboard shelves that I couldn't reach before"

"When I first started doing this—I have a lot of pain with my PD [Parkinson's disease], I have arthritis and I have a lot of issues. I struggle to get up and down the stairs. So I used to get the lift up to my class and the lift down. So about the fourth session I came out of the class and I was chatting away to people and I was at the bottom of the stairs before I realised I had walked down the stairs and I hadn't felt any pain. And it's just the exhilaration of the drumming that had done that"

The benefits of drumming also appeared to have a lasting effect with a positive impact continuing for the rest of the day and a carry-over effect into other activities. Several participants reported improved hand/eye coordination, improved handwriting, and greater amplitude of movement, which they attributed to Parkinson's Beats.

"I am not sure if it is because of the drumming, but I have notice my hand writing has improved recently, and my medication has not changed"

Even though the physical benefits seemed small, they made a big difference. Many reported that they were able to do tasks which they could not do before. Within the focus groups, it became apparent that when they started talking and sharing experiences about how Parkinson's Beats had impacted them, they realised what the changes had been. Enhanced physical and functional benefits were also perceived to fuel changes in mood.

"On drumming days I'm a lot more [chilled] because I don't have the pain and the stiffness"

"I would say, if you want to feel good, and not to feel like you do first thing in the morning, when you need to stretch and it takes half an hour or an hour to get yourself sorted, come to a drumming class. The simple action of using your arms and your hand/eye coordination. It really lifts you body and mind"

3.2. Theme 2. Emotional Impact

Parkinson's Beats was unanimously perceived to have a positive impact on these non-motor symptoms: In terms of immediate impacts, the sessions, participants said, are "Happy" and "It's a happy class". They used the word "euphoria" and noticed that their mood on 'drumming days' was much better than on others:

"Upbeat—you do feel good. You feel up rather than down".

"Parkinson's Beats exercise drumming makes me happy!"

Attending Parkinson's Beats also served as a distraction for many, allowing them to forget about their Parkinson's disease for a period of time:

"Actually doing it, I forget about the Parkinson's"; and "I forget about Parkinson's for the rest of that day".

"It's amazingly relaxing, the whole thing; and you're concentrating on something other than your tremor. You're concentrating on the drumming and forget about your tremor"

Such a distraction appeared to help to mask the daily pain and frustration normally experienced by PLwP. The focus groups all reported that PB drumming helped to reduce stress and improve emotional wellbeing. The impact of music, the act of drumming, and the fun environment created by the instructor were reported as factors which aided the positive impact on the emotional well-being of the group:

"I just love it—it's a selfish thing for me, I love to see people enjoying themselves—it gives so much back to me"

"This is fun—if you can find something you can enjoy then you're more likely to keep it up. She [the instructor] makes it fun, she really does"

Further, a sense of empowerment is also remarked on by participants. Parkinson's Beats promoted "a sense of control", and inclusivity.

"Just enjoy what you can do. Every day is different. Some days you can't do a lot"

"You don't have to—that's the beauty of drumming, you are a free spirit, you do what you like. The more you do it, the better you get as well".

3.3. Theme 3. Impact on Cognitive Function

Participating in Parkinson's Beats presented a cognitive challenge for participants. Participants reported that they enjoyed the challenge of the complex tracks and rhythms:

"I like the more complex [music] tracks" and "There's more for you to do, it's more entertaining, you feel more positive at the end of it"

"You're pushing yourself more as well because some of the more complex movements at more difficult to achieve"

"You have to concentrate so much, and quite a lot of effort put into it".

Participants also found great satisfaction in stretching their skills.

"Pleased with myself, I've accomplished the session" and "Maybe smug would be a better word than content".

However, some participants reported frustrations around balancing between their skills and the challenge of complex tracks and movements:

"That's really important that people don't feel that they have to achieve a standard. Cos there is no standard"

"It just makes me so cross that I can't do it as well as I would like to"

3.4. Theme 4. Social Impact

The participants had a positive experience of being in a group, enjoyment of making music together, and working with others in a group. Parkinson's Beats appeared to have brough a group of PLwP with their limitations all together.

"Trying to finish at the same time as everyone else" and "Being in tune with others is a great feeling"

"The feeling when you're all banging at the same time is great".

"Participants were clear that "Doing it [drumming] on your own wouldn't be the same".

3.5. Theme 5. Additional Benefits

Three subthemes emerged in this theme: music, dance, and the loss of self-consciousness.

Music appears to be the essential impetus for the drumming exercises. Participants felt strongly that they were "Joining in, making [their] own contribution to the track", in effect playing music with the musicians on the recording. "There's something about creating music, dancing to the beat, or drumming to the beat". They are referencing entrainment. The awareness of music permeates the rest of the day, and beyond. "It's funny—I do listen to music in a different way now. I'm thinking: How would I move/beat to that music? you know, when you're in the car, and you bang the steering wheel . . ."

Additionally, some participants incorporated drumming with dancing and movement. The unique blend of uplifting music and aerobic-alike exercises appeared to support dancing and body movements.

"It's more like dancing for me—there's movement in it, and I tend to try to make it into a dance anyway"

Moreover, there were some unexpected benefits for online participants: "I like the zoom. I'm not so sure I'd do it if it wasn't on zoom. I'd be so self-conscious, that I was not hitting the drum at the same time that it would put me off" Offering the Parkinson's Beats sessions online also enabled people to gain benefits: "I like to be able to 'go for it"; "I like being able to lose all of my frustrations"; "Just start making your own noise. Fun. Lash out"; "You can hit the ball as hard as you like".

3.6. Theme 6. Barriers to Participation in Parkinson's Beats

Three potential barriers emerged in the focus group discussions: self-consciousness, retrospection, and the music chosen.

Self-consciousness was overcome through the online setting. One of the online participants said: "I like the zoom. I'm not so sure I'd do it if it wasn't on zoom. I'd be so self-conscious, that I was not hitting the drum at the same time [as the others] that it would put me off".

Another barrier that emerged was raised by a newly diagnosed participant who was frustrated with their own limited mobility and subsequent lack of precision and acknowledged that "I can't forget about my illness when I'm drumming, because it just make me so cross that I can't do it as well as I would like to. [Told, there's no pressure, the participant responded] the pressure is all at my end".

Moreover, a barrier arose for online participants when drumming at home—the impact of the noise on other members of the household. "I have a problem—we now have a rabbit living in the house so now I have to quieten down a bit—the rabbit doesn't like it" and "It can be a problem, the noise. My husband would agree".

Given that part of people's enjoyment of Parkinson's Beats is "I like to be able to 'go for it" and "...lose all of my frustrations" and "making your own noise. Lash out" by hitting the ball "as hard as you like", these restrictions have to be taken into account by the facilitator and the online participants affected.

And finally, the music chosen for the classes was off-putting for some: "A couple of people came but didn't like the music. Said if it was classical, they would be more likely to join".

4. Discussion

This study aimed to explore the perceived impact of cardio-drumming adapted specifically for PLwP using a descriptive phenomenological approach. Six themes and fifteen sub-themes were generated, which highlighted the physical, emotional, cognitive, and social benefits as well as barriers to participating in Parkinson's Beats. It is of interest that some of the perceived benefits were both immediate and lasting over the course of programmes.

Current guidelines recommend a multimodal approach to exercise, encompassing strength, flexibility, balance, and aerobic exercise [37]. The physical benefits reported by participants in Parkinson's Beats may be attributed the fact that drumming combines all these elements within a single workout. Participants also reported perceived improvements in balance following participation in Parkinson's Beats. Improved balance could be attributed to the dual tasking component of Parkinson's Beats whereby drumming rhythmically to the music demands both physical and cognitive resources. Dual tasking involves undertaking two tasks simultaneously: for example, a combination of two motor tasks or a combination of a motor and cognitive task [38]. Several authors have reported that among PLwP the secondary task, regardless of whether it is motor or cognitive, impairs the performance of the primary task [39]. Being able to do two tasks simultaneously is important during many functional tasks such as walking and talking. Consequently, dual task training is advocated in the European Parkinson's Physiotherapy guidelines [40]. A recent systematic review conducted by Beline De Freitas and colleagues [41] demonstrated that dual task training resulted in gait and balance benefits. This study was not designed to explore the effectiveness of Parkinson's Beats on gait and balance, but these perceived benefits may warrant further exploration in a future study.

Additionally, Parkinson's Beats participants reported a range of emotional benefits including enjoyment and the experience of being in a flow. Participants enjoyed having uplifting well-known songs, having the group support, and feeling achievement, as well as being able to 'forget' their Parkinson's during the sessions. These findings were similar to those of previous drumming studies: an in-depth qualitative study involving mental health service users highlighted that the drumming programme appeared to have engendered mental health recovery in the participants [31], as the participants demonstrated enhanced enjoyment, agency, accomplishments, engagement, and positive self-identity [31]. In particular, the Parkinson's Beats study participants also reported experiences of being in a flow, which is characterised by being totally immersed in the joy of the activity; this experience of being in a flow has been conceptualised by Csikszentmihalyi [42,43]. Being in a flow can be highly motivational, as we experience heightened enjoyment of an activity that balances challenge and stretches our ability to meet and surpass those challenges [42,43]. This is evident in our study participants, PLwP, who were motivated by their sense of happiness, exhilaration, and outright euphoria. Similar findings were reported in an African drumming study involving older adults (N = 27) with dementia, who showed improvements in mood, level of interest, responsiveness, engagement, and enjoyment [26]. In another controlled study, a three-month Japanese drumming exercise programme resulted in reduced depressive mood and improved physical fitness in community-dwelling older women ($\geq$65 years) (N = 40) [44]. Further, a randomised controlled study demonstrated significantly reduced depression and anxiety and increased wellbeing and social resilience in the drumming group participants compared with the control group [30]. This study also tested participants' saliva samples and found that drumming resulted in increases in anti-inflammatory activity [30].

Moreover, a sense of empowerment was also remarked on by Parkinson's Beats participants. Empowerment is variously described as "a process whereby people gain mastery over their affairs" [45]; "helping patients discover and develop inherent capacity to be responsible for one's own life" [46]; and a sense of power and control of one's condition. Rawlet [47] proposes that empowerment is determined by one's self-efficacy. Levels of empowerment are associated with levels of quality of life: when PLwP have the capacity to control their own management and take personal responsibility for their own well-being, this can be empowering and yields an enhanced quality of life despite the seemingly limiting condition [48].

Due to Parkinson's, coordinating one's movements becomes increasingly difficult; however, Parkinson's Beats participants reported improved skills and concentration (Theme 3). With the help of strong beats in the accompanying songs, the participants perceived there were benefits for the brain. Such cognitive benefits were evident in a 15-week controlled drumming study with older adults (N = 24), who felt their cognitive functions were declining [49]. This study was designed to progress from simple tasks to more complex tasks including drumming and singing for older adults. After the 15-week programme, the drumming group participants demonstrated improved visual memory compared with the literary control group. Thus, this study indicated that drumming programmes can potentially prevent cognitive declining [49].

Moreover, Parkinson's Beats is inclusive because the exercises can be adapted to accommodate individual limitations and capacities. For example, PLwP can use one arm or two, be standing or seated; most will drum in real time, but the beat can be slowed to half time for anyone finding difficulty with the speed and frequency of the rhythm. Each session was led by an experienced facilitator who created an atmosphere of trust and safety, enabling participants to become free to express themselves, and enjoy themselves. The facilitator demonstrated enthusiasm and provided encouragement throughout the sessions. Additionally, our study demonstrated that Parkinson's Beats can be delivered both face to face and online, where participants' experiences were similar, although in some cases, the online format was preferred due to the option of not being seen/heard, which helped overcome self-consciousness. However, online participation, i.e., drumming at home may require some pre-arrangements with family members, who may not enjoy the noise. Further, the facilitators are required to have sound knowledge and understanding of Parkinson's and its progressive impacts on participants. As we highlighted in Theme 6, the facilitator may need to provide extra support for those who are newly diagnosed, as the newly diagnosed participants may experience much frustration when they face their own limited mobility and subsequent lack of precision during drumming. Finally, collaborating on the song choices with participants could minimise disappointment or disagreement, as well as encourage participants to take ownership.

Limitations and Strengths

This study was an exploratory pilot research study, which highlighted the experiences of PLwP who participated in cardio-drumming exercises. This study is based on responses of 19 participants who were interviewed in three focus groups. Arguably, a larger sample size could potentially yield richer data; however, the sample size in the current study aligns with prior Parkinson's qualitative research. Guest, Bunce, and Johnson [50] found that across a sample size of sixty interviews, category saturation occurred within the first twelve interviews and that the basic elements for core themes were present within the first six interviews. Therefore, the data gathered from 19 participants in the current study were regarded as sufficient for the purpose of this study.

Further, we acknowledge that the researchers conducting the focus groups (AW and JH) have experience of drumming and they themselves live with Parkinson's. While this may have the potential to introduce bias, the fact that they have lived experience of Parkinson's may have allowed the collection of richer data, as participants may have felt more at ease during the focus groups. While the use of researchers who have Parkinson's may have introduced some bias, this was mitigated during the data analysis, which was conducted by all members of the research team.

5. Conclusions

The findings of Parkinson's Beats, a cardio-drumming exercise programme for people living with Parkinson's (PLwP), has demonstrated physical, emotional, cognitive, and social benefits. PLwP reported enhanced mobility and reach, as well as reduced stiffness and pain. A range of positive feelings were evident, including feeling euphoric, uplifted, and joyful. Additionally, participants experienced flow and empowerment. Group sessions also enhanced social wellbeing. Future studies may include physical, cognitive, and psychological assessments, and investigate both short-term and long-term impacts, with appropriate comparators (e.g., other types of physical activities, online vs in-person delivery, healthy controls). Research into the optimal dose of cardio-drumming for different stages of Parkinson's progression is also needed. Moreover, best practice guidelines for the facilitators/instructors on how to deliver a cardio-drumming exercise programme tailored for PLwP need to be developed using evidence-based research. Further research should also explore the possibility of Parkinson's Beats being prescribed as an integral part of the personalised health plans of PLwP.

Author Contributions: Conceptualisation and investigation: J.J., J.Y.I., J.H. and A.W.; data analysis: A.W. and J.H.; writing: J.Y.I., A.W. and J.J.; funding acquisition: J.J., J.Y.I., J.H. and A.W. All authors have read and agreed to the published version of the manuscript.

Funding: This research was funded by the Parkinson's UK Excellence Network UK (215 Vauxhall Bridge Road, London, SW1V 1EJ), grant number M-22-002.

Institutional Review Board Statement: The study was conducted in accordance with the Declaration of Helsinki and was reviewed and approved by the Research Ethics Committee, School of Health Science, Robert Gordon University, UK (Reference number: SREC SHS/22/32, received on 7 December 2022).

Informed Consent Statement: Informed consent was obtained from all participants involved.

Data Availability Statement: The data are not publicly available due to ethical restrictions. The data can be obtained from the corresponding author based on a reasonable request for research purposes.

Acknowledgments: The authors would like to thank all participants that contributed to this research, and the reviewers for their positive and constructive comments and suggestions.

Conflicts of Interest: The authors declare no conflicts of interest.

References

1. Collaborator Group. Global, regional, and national burden of neurological disorders during 1990–2015: A systematic analysis for the Global Burden of Disease Study 2015. *Lancet Neurol.* **2017**, *16*, 877–897. [CrossRef] [PubMed]
2. Ou, Z.; Pan, J.; Tang, S.; Duan, D.; Yu, D.; Nong, H.; Wang, Z. Global Trends in the Incidence, Prevalence, and Years Lived With Disability of Parkinson's Disease in 204 Countries/Territories From 1990 to 2019. *Front. Public Health.* **2021**, *7*, 776847. [CrossRef] [PubMed]
3. Zhao, A.; Cui, E.; Leroux, A.; Lindquist, M.A.; Crainiceanu, C.M. Evaluating the prediction performance of objective physical activity measures for incident Parkinson's disease in the UK Biobank. *J. Neurol.* **2023**, *270*, 5913–5923. [CrossRef] [PubMed]
4. Bloem, B.R.; Okun, M.S.; Klein, C. Parkinson's disease. *Lancet* **2021**, *397*, 2284–2303. [CrossRef] [PubMed]
5. Kalia, L.V.; Lang, A.E. Parkinson's disease. *Lancet* **2015**, *29*, 896–912. [CrossRef] [PubMed]
6. Chaudhuri, K.R.; Naidu, Y. Early Parkinson's disease and non-motor issues. *J. Neurol.* **2008**, *255* (Suppl. S5), 33–38. [CrossRef] [PubMed]
7. Poewe, W.; Mahlknecht, P. The clinical progression of Parkinson's disease. *Park. Relat. Disord.* **2009**, *15* (Suppl. S4), S28–S32. [CrossRef] [PubMed]
8. Ferrazzoli, D.; Ortelli, P.; Zivi, I.; Cian, V.; Urso, E.; Ghilardi, M.F.; Maestri, R.; Frazzitta, G. Efficacy of intensive multidisciplinary rehabilitation in Parkinson's disease: A randomised controlled study. *J. Neurol. Neurosurg. Psychiatry* **2018**, *89*, 828–835. [CrossRef] [PubMed]
9. Hechtner, M.C.; Vogt, T.; Zöllner, Y.; Schröder, S.; Sauer, J.B.; Binder, H.; Singer, S.; Mikolajczyk, R. Quality of life in Parkinson's disease patients with motor fluctuations and dyskinesias in five European countries. *Park. Relat. Disord.* **2014**, *20*, 969–974. [CrossRef] [PubMed]
10. Chen, H.; Zhang, S.M.; Schwarzschild, M.A.; Hernán, M.A.; Ascherio, A. Physical activity and the risk of Parkinson disease. *Neurology* **2005**, *22*, 664–669. [CrossRef]
11. Hirsch, M.A.; Iyer, S.S.; Sanjak, M. Exercise-induced neuroplasticity in human Parkinson's disease: What is the evidence telling us? *Park. Relat. Disord.* **2016**, *22* (Suppl. S1), S78–S81. [CrossRef] [PubMed]
12. Johansson, M.E.; Cameron, I.G.M.; Van der Kolk, N.M.; de Vries, N.M.; Klimars, E.; Toni, I.; Bloem, B.R.; Helmich, R.C. Aerobic Exercise Alters Brain Function and Structure in Parkinson's Disease: A Randomized Controlled Trial. *Ann. Neurol.* **2022**, *91*, 203–216. [CrossRef]
13. Yitayeh, A.; Teshome, A. The effectiveness of physiotherapy treatment on balance dysfunction and postural instability in persons with Parkinson's disease: A systematic review and meta-analysis. *BMC Sports Sci. Med. Rehabil.* **2016**, *8*, 17. [CrossRef] [PubMed]
14. Paolucci, T.; Sbardella, S.; La Russa, C.; Agostini, F.; Mangone, M.; Tramontana, L.; Bernetti, A.; Paoloni, M.; Pezzi, L.; Bellomo, R.G.; et al. Evidence of Rehabilitative Impact of Progressive Resistance Training (PRT) Programs in Parkinson Disease: An Umbrella Review. *Park. Dis.* **2020**, *2020*, 9748091. [CrossRef] [PubMed]
15. de Almeida, F.O.; Santana, V.; Corcos, D.M.; Ugrinowitsch, C.; Silva-Batista, C. Effects of Endurance Training on Motor Signs of Parkinson's Disease: A Systematic Review and Meta-Analysis. *Sports Med.* **2022**, *52*, 1789–1815. [CrossRef] [PubMed]
16. Gamborg, M.; Hvid, L.G.; Dalgas, U.; Langeskov-Christensen, M. Parkinson's disease and intensive exercise therapy—An updated systematic review and meta-analysis. *Acta Neurol. Scand.* **2022**, *145*, 504–528. [CrossRef] [PubMed]
17. Cusso, M.E.; Donald, K.J.; Khoo, T.K. The Impact of Physical Activity on Non-Motor Symptoms in Parkinson's Disease: A Systematic Review. *Front. Med.* **2016**, *3*, 35. [CrossRef] [PubMed]
18. Ramazzina, I.; Bernazzoli, B.; Costantino, C. Systematic review on strength training in Parkinson's disease: An unsolved question. *Clin. Interv. Aging* **2017**, *31*, 619–628. [CrossRef]
19. Wu, P.L.; Lee, M.; Huang, T.T. Effectiveness of physical activity on patients with depression and Parkinson's disease: A systematic review. *PLoS ONE* **2017**, *12*, e0181515. [CrossRef]
20. da Silva, F.C.; Iop, R.D.R.; de Oliveira, L.C.; Boll, A.M.; de Alvarenga, J.G.S.; Gutierres Filho, P.J.B.; de Melo, L.M.A.B.; Xavier, A.J.; da Silva, R. Effects of physical exercise programs on cognitive function in Parkinson's disease patients: A systematic review of randomized controlled trials of the last 10 years. *PLoS ONE* **2018**, *13*, e0193113. [CrossRef]
21. Chen, K.; Tan, Y.; Lu, Y.; Wu, J.; Liu, X.; Zhao, Y. Effect of Exercise on Quality of Life in Parkinson's Disease: A Systematic Review and Meta-Analysis. *Park. Dis.* **2020**, *2020*, 3257623. [CrossRef] [PubMed]
22. Cristini, J.; Weiss, M.; De Las Heras, B.; Medina-Rincón, A.; Dagher, A.; Postuma, R.B.; Huber, R.; Doyon, J.; Rosa-Neto, P.; Carrier, J.; et al. The effects of exercise on sleep quality in persons with Parkinson's disease: A systematic review with meta-analysis. *Sleep Med. Rev.* **2021**, *55*, 101384. [CrossRef] [PubMed]
23. Radder, D.L.M.; Lígia Silva de Lima, A.; Domingos, J.; Keus, S.H.J.; van Nimwegen, M.; Bloem, B.R.; de Vries, N.M. Physiotherapy in Parkinson's Disease: A Meta-Analysis of Present Treatment Modalities. *Neurorehabil. Neural Repair* **2020**, *34*, 871–880. [CrossRef] [PubMed]
24. De La Rue, S.E.; Draper, S.B.; Potter, C.R.; Smith, M.S. Energy expenditure in rock/pop drumming. *Int. J. Sports Med.* **2013**, *34*, 868–872. [CrossRef] [PubMed]
25. Stern, C. Break it down! Viral Video Shows Senior Citizens in a D'Rum Fitness Class' Banging on Exercise Balls to the Beat of Bruno Mars' Uptown Funk. Daily Mail Newspaper. 2021. Available online: https://www.dailymail.co.uk/femail/article-9216551/Viral-video-shows-seniors-nursing-home-drumming-exercise-balls-tune-Uptown-Funk.html (accessed on 5 April 2023).

26. Roy, M.; Devroop, K.; Bohn, A. The Positive Impact of African Drumming on Elderly Participants' Mood and Demeanour. *Muziki* **2019**, *16*, 113–125. [CrossRef]
27. Thaut, M.H.; McIntosh, G.C.; Hoemberg, V. Neurobiological foundations of neurologic music therapy: Rhythmic entrainment and the motor system. *Front. Psychol.* **2015**, *5*, 1185. [CrossRef] [PubMed]
28. Schaffert, N.; Janzen, T.B.; Mattes, K.; Thaut, M.H. A Review on the Relationship Between Sound and Movement in Sports and Rehabilitation. *Front. Psychol.* **2019**, *10*, 244. [CrossRef] [PubMed]
29. de Dreu, M.J.; van der Wilk, A.S.; Poppe, E.; Kwakkel, G.; van Wegen, E.E. Rehabilitation, exercise therapy and music in patients with Parkinson's disease: A meta-analysis of the effects of music-based movement therapy on walking ability, balance and quality of life. *Park. Relat. Disord.* **2012**, *18* (Suppl. S1), S114–S119. [CrossRef]
30. Fancourt, D.; Perkins, R.; Ascenso, S.; Carvalho, L.A.; Steptoe, A.; Williamon, A. Effects of Group Drumming Interventions on Anxiety, Depression, Social Resilience and Inflammatory Immune Response among Mental Health Service Users. *PLoS ONE* **2016**, *11*, e0151136. [CrossRef]
31. Ascenso, S.; Perkins, R.; Atkins, L.; Fancourt, D.; Williamon, A. Promoting well-being through group drumming with mental health service users and their carers. *Int. J. Qual. Stud. Health Well-Being* **2018**, *13*, 1484219. [CrossRef]
32. Pantelyat, A.; Syres, C.; Reichwein, S.; Willis, A. DRUM-PD: The use of a drum circle to improve the symptoms and signs of Parkinson's disease (PD). *Mov. Disord. Clin. Pract.* **2016**, *3*, 243–249. [CrossRef] [PubMed]
33. Sundler, A.J.; Lindberg, E.; Nilsson, C.; Palmér, L. Qualitative thematic analysis based on descriptive phenomenology. *Nurs. Open* **2019**, *6*, 733–739. [CrossRef] [PubMed]
34. Spencer, L.; Ritchie, J.; Lewis, J.; Dillon, L. Quality in Qualitative Evaluation: A Framework for Assessing Research Evidence. 2003. Available online: https://assets.publishing.service.gov.uk/media/5a8179c1ed915d74e33fe69e/Quality-in-qualitative-evaulation_tcm6-38739.pdf (accessed on 5 April 2023).
35. Ritchie, J.; Lewis, J.; Nicholls, C.M.; Ormston, R. (Eds.) *Qualitative Research Practice: A Guide for Social Science Students and Researchers*; Sage: Thousand Oaks, CA, USA, 2013.
36. Gale, N.K.; Heath, G.; Cameron, E.; Rashid, S.; Redwood, S. Using the framework method for the analysis of qualitative data in multi-disciplinary health research. *BMC Med. Res. Methodol.* **2013**, *13*, 117. [CrossRef] [PubMed]
37. Osborne, J.A.; Botkin, R.; Colon-Semenza, C.; DeAngelis, T.R.; Gallardo, O.G.; Kosakowski, H.; Martello, J.; Pradhan, S.; Rafferty, M.; Readinger, J.L.; et al. Physical Therapist Management of Parkinson Disease: A Clinical Practice Guideline From the American Physical Therapy Association. *Phys. Ther.* **2022**, *102*, pzab302, Erratum in *Phys. Ther.* **2022**, *102*, pzac098. [CrossRef] [PubMed]
38. Broeder, S.; Nackaerts, E.; Nieuwboer, A.; Smits-Engelsman, B.C.; Swinnen, S.P.; Heremans, E. The effects of dual tasking on handwriting in patients with Parkinson's disease. *Neuroscience* **2014**, *263*, 193–202. [CrossRef]
39. Rochester, L.; Galna, B.; Lord, S.; Burn, D. The nature of dual-task interference during gait in incident Parkinson's disease. *Neuroscience* **2014**, *265*, 83–94. [CrossRef] [PubMed]
40. Domingos, J.; Keus, S.H.J.; Dean, J.; de Vries, N.M.; Ferreira, J.J.; Bloem, B.R. The European Physiotherapy Guideline for Parkinson's Disease: Implications for Neurologists. *J. Park. Dis.* **2018**, *8*, 499–502. [CrossRef] [PubMed]
41. De Freitas, T.B.; Leite, P.H.W.; Doná, F.; Pompeu, J.E.; Swarowsky, A.; Torriani-Pasin, C. The effects of dual task gait and balance training in Parkinson's disease: A systematic review. *Physiother. Theory Pract.* **2020**, *36*, 1088–1096. [CrossRef] [PubMed]
42. Csikszentmihalyi, M. *Beyond Boredom and Anxiety*; Jossey-Bass: Hoboken, NJ, USA, 2000.
43. Csíkszentmihályi, M.; Csíkszentmihályi, I.S. (Eds.) *Optimal Experience: Psychological Studies of Flow in Consciousness*; Cambridge University Press: Cambridge, UK, 1988; pp. 15–35. [CrossRef]
44. Tanaka, M.; Komura, F.; Hanai, A.; Tsuboyama, T.; Arai, H. Effects of Japanese drum exercise on depression and physical function in community-dwelling older women. *J. Clin. Gerontol. Geriatr.* **2016**, *7*, 158–163. [CrossRef]
45. Rappaport, J. Terms of empowerment/exemplars of prevention: Toward a theory for community psychology. *Am. J. Community Psychol.* **1987**, *15*, 121–148. [CrossRef]
46. Funnell, M.M.; Anderson, R.M.; Arnold, M.S.; Barr, P.A.; Donnelly, M.; Johnson, P.D.; Taylor-Moon, D.; White, N.H. Empowerment: An idea whose time has come in diabetes education. *Diabetes Educ.* **1991**, *17*, 37–41. [CrossRef] [PubMed]
47. Rawlett, K.E. Journey from self-efficacy to empowerment. *Health Care* **2014**, *2*, 1–9. [CrossRef]
48. Williams, A.; Jones, J. Supporting the Journey to Empowerment for People with Parkinson's through the Person-Centred Lens of Those Living with Parkinson's. Edinburgh Parkinson's. 2023. Available online: https://www.edinburghparkinsons.org/wp-content/uploads/2023/03/Williams-and-Jones-article.pdf (accessed on 5 April 2023).
49. Degé, F.; Kerkovius, K. The effects of drumming on working memory in older adults. *Ann. N. Y. Acad. Sci.* **2018**, *1423*, 242–250. [CrossRef] [PubMed]
50. Guest, G.; Bunce, A.; Johnson, L. How Many Interviews Are Enough?: An Experiment with Data Saturation and Variability. *Field Methods* **2006**, *18*, 59–82. [CrossRef]

Disclaimer/Publisher's Note: The statements, opinions and data contained in all publications are solely those of the individual author(s) and contributor(s) and not of MDPI and/or the editor(s). MDPI and/or the editor(s) disclaim responsibility for any injury to people or property resulting from any ideas, methods, instructions or products referred to in the content.

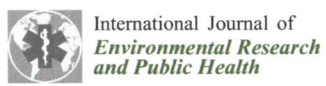

Review

"We Can Do This!": The Role of Physical Activity in What Comes Next for Dementia

Christopher Russell

Association for Dementia Studies, University of Worcester, Henwick Grove, Worcester WR2 6AJ, UK; c.russell@worc.ac.uk

Abstract: There is increasing interest in physical activity as a response to the harm caused by dementia. The focus has been upon interventions to prevent or delay symptoms or to support people living with the condition to reminisce. Whilst this is welcome, there are other features inherent to physical activity that remain unrecognised or underutilised and, consequently, its full potential for good is unrealised. Most prominent is the ability physical activity has to enable participants to claim and sustain a place in the world through what they do, crucial to a context where the impact of dementia tends to annihilate this for those living with the condition. The article addresses this gap. In doing so, it presents key findings. These include (1) highlighting the fundamental importance of features such as person-centred care, human rights and social citizenship to enabling people with dementia to live lives of quality and (2) identifying synergies with these features and what physical activity can offer; for example, emphasising the value of bringing these together to illustrate how physical activity can contribute to enabling people with dementia to live lives characterised by quality, and the maintenance of their place in the world. The article concludes by suggesting what must come next to ensure physical activity can play the fullest role possible.

Keywords: dementia; physical activity; person-centred; human rights; citizenship; relationships; agency; power; the everyday; leisure

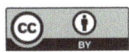

Citation: Russell, C. "We Can Do This!": The Role of Physical Activity in What Comes Next for Dementia. *Int. J. Environ. Res. Public Health* **2023**, *20*, 6503. https://doi.org/10.3390/ijerph20156503

Academic Editors: Andy Pringle, Nicola Kime and Gregory W. Heath

Received: 4 May 2023
Revised: 6 July 2023
Accepted: 27 July 2023
Published: 2 August 2023

Copyright: © 2023 by the author. Licensee MDPI, Basel, Switzerland. This article is an open access article distributed under the terms and conditions of the Creative Commons Attribution (CC BY) license (https://creativecommons.org/licenses/by/4.0/).

1. Introduction

This article focuses upon life with dementia and the role physical activity should play within it. It highlights how modern thinking about dementia (in particular, two dementia-related paradigms: person-centred care and support and social citizenship) aligns with insights garnered from contemporary scholarship about physical activity. Insight into this modern thinking is offered to illustrate ways in which physical activity can offer much to people living with dementia beyond improvements to physical health (important though these are) and how physical activity can contribute to enabling people with dementia to sustain their place in the world. Suggestions are made so that practice can be tailored to maximise the benefits such approaches can bring, and the article concludes by highlighting key areas for attention so progress can be realised. Firstly, however, dementia and physical activity are explained alongside a fuller rationale for what follows.

Dementia is an umbrella term used to describe a number of diseases or conditions that cause irreversible damage to the brain, with symptoms that inevitably progress over time. The nature of these will vary depending on the particular form of dementia causing illness; for example, Alzheimer's disease (the most common form of dementia) is characterised by memory loss in relation to contemporary events [1,2]. Only very recently has any advancement been made with pharmacological interventions that might alter the progression of symptoms [3]. Possible breakthroughs relate solely to Alzheimer's disease and are limited to intervention at early stages of the illness, with delivery available through intense and uncomfortable means (i.e., subcutaneously). The potential for malign side effects means that, in large parts of the world, regulatory bodies remain reluctant to approve use [4,5].

The fact that pharmacology has been unable to offer definitive responses to dementia has caused concern for individuals living with dementia, their families and health and care professionals [6]. In part, this is because, as symptoms progress, the ability of people to continue to play an agentic role in everyday life is corroded and eventually destroyed [7]. In addition, dementia is universally feared because of the impact it can have upon an individual's sense of self and identity [6,8], with those living with the condition reporting feelings of stigmatisation and low self-esteem [9]. These matters, allied to the fact that very large numbers of people across the world are living with dementia or predicted to be living with it over the next fifty years [10], have made dementia a global public health priority [11].

With this context to the fore, research and scholarship have sought to comprehend best practice in areas related to the provision of care and support for people affected by dementia [12]. This has given rise to concepts characterised as "psycho-social" approaches. These include person-centred care [6] and personhood [8], which can contribute to enabling people with dementia to live lives characterised by quality by encouraging others to attend to individual need and maximising the quality of relationships inherent to the daily life of the person [13]. In recent times, these approaches have increasingly been regarded as inadequate in themselves because of the risk that they may foreground people living with dementia as patients rather than whole people, solely with needs to be met rather than lives to be led [14]. Critique has been driven, in large part, by people living with dementia, who, in the last 10 years or so, have advocated for enhanced recognition of the role of human rights in any discourse about dementia [15]. This has drawn upon, and simultaneously fuelled, an increasingly influential paradigm espousing social citizenship in dementia [16].

Citizenship is a comprehensive and complex phenomenon, the subject of study and interpretation over many years [17]. This dynamism is part of it, with rights and responsibilities of individuals and those of the state renegotiated as contemporary societal circumstances change [17]. In fact, defining citizenship should not be easy because such vitality of meaning is what enables it to be effective [18]. Social citizenship is the interpretation that has been adopted within the dementia context. It is a relationship or practice (as much as a status) whereby an individual living with dementia must feel free from discrimination and have opportunities to grow and participate in life as fully as possible [16]. Social citizenship involves the upholding of rights, with international frameworks—such as Article 30 of the United Nation's Convention on the Rights of Persons with Disabilities—being seminal in enabling an authoritative rather than optional status [19]. Allied to this modern thinking is the necessity that people living with dementia should expect every actor with influence in their daily life (ranging from shop keepers to surgeons, depending on prevailing circumstances) to offer opportunities for the fullest engagement possible in "everyday life". The nature of "everyday life" is seen as fundamental to social citizenship, with the mundane components of the everyday being the context in which people living with dementia manifest their ongoing place in the world [17].

Physical activity is defined as any intentional movement produced by the skeletal muscles that results in increased energy expenditure [20]. The broad nature of this interpretation means it is capable of being part of everyday life. Sadly, however, physical activity is not routinely on offer to people living with dementia [21]. There are many reasons for this, with one of the most prominent being that knowledge of what works well in terms of the provision of physical activity is limited [22]. However, as will be shown, physical activity is well placed to align with contemporary thinking about dementia because it can be used to harness elements of person-centred support and contribute to the social citizenship of people living with dementia. For these reasons, it should, therefore, be included as a fundamental part of the ongoing response to dementia.

2. Responses to Dementia and the Part Played by Physical Activity

There is increasing and global interest in what physical activity can offer to people living with dementia [23] because of its contributions in several different ways; for example, via potentially averting, holding up or improving symptoms of dementia [24,25], with evidence that suitable interventions may slacken the rate of disease progression [26]. In addition, within the field of dementia reminiscence, physical activity has been employed to stimulate memories of times past in the lives of individuals; for example, through use of Irish dancing [27]. However, what is proposed here, a focus upon person-centred and social citizenship approaches in dementia, builds upon and moves beyond this by highlighting how additional benefit can be realised through physical activity supporting and promoting one's place in the world or in the everyday lives of participants with dementia. Furthermore, such understanding will enable those offering opportunities for physical activity to tailor what they do to enhance its ability to contribute even more than it already does, this being especially important because of the lack of reliable and accessible pharmacological responses to dementia. In the following paragraphs, therefore, person-centred and citizen approaches are explained in detail. Key aspects are identified that, as will be indicated, hold relevance for those interested in adapting approaches to physical activity for individuals living with dementia.

Turning first to person-centred support, over the last 25 years, there has been a move from considerations of dementia as primarily a medical condition to something recognised as affecting all aspects of a person's experience of life [8]. Fundamental is the fact that, as every person is unique, everybody's experience of dementia is different. Taking a person-centred approach therefore means ensuring that everyone living with dementia is recognised in terms of their life story, abilities and skills, personality and physical health rather than being defined only by the damage to cognition caused by dementia [6,12]. Furthermore, to facilitate person-centred approaches to care and support, what is known as "personhood" must be promoted. This is defined as "a standing or status that is bestowed upon one human being, by others, in the context of relationship and social being. It implies recognition, respect and trust" ([8], p. 8). Thus, the relationships an individual living with dementia has with others and the quality of those relationships in terms of enabling that person to sustain their feeling of self and identity matter. If these are not of sufficient quality, person-centred support cannot be sustained.

For the best part of a quarter of a century these ideas have formed the foundations of approaches to care and support in dementia [6]. However, person-centred approaches alone are insufficient to enable people with dementia to live lives of quality [14]. Emphasis by clinical services upon earlier diagnosis [28] has enabled more people living with dementia to articulate what matters to them in everyday life [29]. Through accounts of people themselves, and via allied research and scholarship, has come the call for human rights and social citizenship to be prioritised in ways not represented within person-centred approaches. For example, Bartlett and O'Connor [14], writing in 2007, highlighted that the structural nature of societies and the agency held by people living with dementia also needed to be taken into account. Thus, people living with dementia should be recognised as individuals whose experience of life is informed by their gender, class, ethnicity, sexuality, ability, and age [17].

A focus upon human rights is required because person-centred approaches alone fail to affirm the ongoing status of people as having power to influence their lives [30]. This, in turn, highlights the need to promote the ongoing place in the world of people living with dementia as citizens [17]. All too often, people lack agency [31] or indeed opportunity to demonstrate this, and later it will be argued that physical activity is well positioned to redress this. However, before addressing this directly, more detail is required relating to the nature of citizenship approaches in the context of dementia. This concerns elements that contribute to the foundations of this article's core argument: that modern thinking about dementia (aligned with insights garnered from contemporary scholarship about physical activity) illustrates how physical activity can contribute to enabling people with dementia to live lives characterised by quality and sustain their place in the world.

Firstly, the nature of everyday life with dementia is now viewed as crucial. This is because it is here that the practical conditions for the participation and influence of individuals occur [17]. Thus, as Nedlund and colleagues advocated in 2019 [17], there is a need to take the ordinary seriously. Furthermore, as Butchard and Dunne [29] point out, the human rights of people living with dementia are liable to violation on an everyday basis. The example they highlight is the "task-driven" nature of care, removing the opportunities many people living with dementia have to influence what goes on or to express their preferences. Instead, social citizenship approaches advocate that people living with dementia should be enabled to explain or demonstrate what they wish to happen on an everyday basis and thus enact their human rights. As will be suggested later, physical activity provides a unique ability for individuals living with dementia to demonstrate this.

Secondly, the quality of relationships matters in ways extending beyond those identified within person-centred support. So, for example, Sabat [32] argued there should be no "us" and "them" when considering life with dementia. He advocated for approaches supportive of "shared humanity" ([32], p. 12). This theme has been built upon [17] with the suggestion that citizenship-based relationships should foster feelings of belonging, with a focus upon recognition of shared experiences within communal care settings, for example. Other people play a significant role in affirming the integrity of self-worth for people living with dementia through their actions and behaviour towards them [33]. Thus, those people, key within the lives of each individual, can contribute to the citizenship of a person through relationships characterised by shared humanity, a sense of belonging and affirmation of an individual's self-worth [17,32,33].

How this might occur is related to a third point, which is that, in terms of recognition, it is acknowledgement by others of the agency held by the person living with dementia that matters most [34]. This is congruent with a "strengths-based approach" [32] in the dementia context, which prioritises abilities a person retains rather than those they may have lost as a result of the illness. Nedlund and colleagues [17] characterised this as shifting the focus from that exclusively upon care towards understanding that people can and must retain power. This should pertain to people at an advanced stage of dementia too and in such circumstances can be manifested via displays of "embodied agency" [34], where people employ actions to express their will if no longer able to do so verbally. As a result of the harm caused by advanced dementia, these can be subtle movements or gestures offered by individuals through what have been described as "micro-gestures" [17]. Those who may be supporting people with advanced dementia (for example, paid or family carers) must assist them by knowing them well and being able to understand their significance. This is "relational citizenship" [35], where individuals use their bodies to express their place in the world. The opportunities afforded for this by physical activity are clear. Unlike other leisure-based activities, such as singing or art, which potentially afford similar benefits in terms of communality and presence to people living with dementia, physical activity uniquely and by its very nature offers opportunity for individuals to employ their bodies to achieve such constructive outcomes. It is noteworthy also that relational citizenship in the dementia context is based upon the premise that people must be active partners in their own care. Thus, agency, power and how these are manifested by individuals and recognised by others form cornerstones of modern approaches to citizenship in dementia.

A rights- and citizenship-based approach is founded upon ethical concerns for social justice, fairness and equality. With regard to dementia, this has been described as "a discourse of hope" ([30], p. 18). That physical activity has a key role to play enhancing the social citizenship of people living with dementia is, therefore, exciting and positive. With these factors in mind, and drawing upon the discussion so far, the article now turns to the role of physical activity in everyday life with dementia.

3. The Role of Physical Activity in Everyday Life with Dementia

Physical activity is an inextricable part of the everyday. This is reflected in numerous studies exploring physical activity in the context of life with dementia (as will be shown below). Thus, it is well placed to form an essential part of the response to the condition. For example, a study by Olsen and colleagues in 2015 [36], which had as its basis a high-intensity functional exercise programme for those with dementia living in a nursing home, found there was much participants valued related to the everyday. Thus, individuals reported that participation enabled them to feel "...more like a normal person" ([36], p. 6). This was related to physical activity having felt relevant to the everyday life of participants throughout earlier times and this feeling extending into daily living within the context of the nursing home; for example, enhancing one's energy to engage within social discourse and offering the chance for such opportunities to happen in the first place via the provision of the physical activity. Writing in 2022, Telenius and colleagues [37] highlighted similar features. Their study involved interviews with people living with dementia to explore their experience of physical activity. Notable here were participant reflections about physical activity giving content and structure to their days. "Everyday" activities, such as mowing the grass, were highlighted as examples. The significance of the seemingly mundane had deeper consequences, however, when considered against what was discussed about agency and power. Participants noted, for example, that such routines enabled them to exert feelings of control within daily life that would otherwise be missing.

Of course, what individuals choose to do with the everyday must not be prescribed. This article champions person-centred approaches based upon rights and citizenship within everyday contexts, and people not only have a right to choose what they do in later life but they also have the right to choose to do nothing very active if this is their wish [38]. However, because physical activity is so diverse in nature, it is well placed to embrace a range of activities that may align with the preferences individuals have for activity in their everyday lives. A study by Burke and Jones [39] is illustrative. It focused upon experiences of people living with dementia within sheltered housing and care homes but, unlike the research conducted by Olsen et al. [36], investigated reflections offered by participants engaging in "low threshold" sports programmes. This placed "minimal demands" ([39], p. 2) in terms of what was required or expected of individuals. Facilitators were not themselves highly trained sports professionals or therapists; instead, they were provided with training in the interventions in order to offer them with confidence. Participants enjoyed what they did, and it was noted that provision could be sustained over the long term because it was "open to all" and sociable in nature. This low-threshold physical activity had the potential to act as a gateway to further opportunities for individuals ([39], p. 8).

Thus, physical activity has an important role to play in what is on offer to people living with dementia as part of everyday life, bringing benefits in terms of sustaining an individual's place in the world through what they do and experience. Other studies have affirmed this, including that by Hartfiel et al. [26], which, although investigating outcomes of an organised exercise programme for people living with dementia, highlighted how the formation of habits revolving around physical activity was beneficial for individuals. For example, one participant reported that, after engaging in the programme, he had gone on to complete nearly 40 park runs. The everyday is about tailoring physical activity to what is relevant to the person living with dementia [24]. This can be highly structured and organised or it can be as mundane as shovelling snow [36]. Links here to the earlier discussion about the need to pay attention to person-centred approaches are clear.

The nature and quality of relationships held by people living with dementia were identified (above) as positive and fundamental in enabling individuals to sustain their place in the world. Physical activity has been shown to offer opportunity for such constructive relationships. For example, Olsen and colleagues [36] found that it was the interactions amongst participants that contributed significantly to those individuals realising the outcomes they wished to achieve from the activity, here acting as role models for each other, demonstrating what was possible and motivating each other to participate. As one respondent said: "...we can do this!" ([36], p. 6). Collaboration is seen as a powerful and positive enabler in sustaining one's place in the world in the context of life with dementia [17,33]. This involves not only a sense of belonging, which, as has already been highlighted, is key to the sort of empowerment at the heart of this discussion, but also feelings of agency and of holding power in relation to what is being enacted. Confidence to engage in such collaborative actions can come from within the group itself [26]. However, there are nuances and skills that facilitators must be aware of in order to foster collaboration. These include the willingness of those nominally charged with providing physical activity to enable participants living with dementia to lead and facilitate such activity at times or throughout the process, if this is their wish [24]. The provision of physical activity in such ways can have beneficial outcomes for staff and volunteers too; for example, increased optimism and positivity have been reported throughout settings where this has taken place [24]. When this operates successfully, encounters by those living with dementia with staff have been found to be characterised by vitality rather than detachment [36]. These are important attributes linked to the provision of physical activity within a context where so often the wellbeing and motivation of the dementia care workforce is not found to be so buoyant [40,41].

This discussion has shown that physical activity can act as an enabler of agency and power for people living with dementia. The significance of this to the facilitation of an ongoing sense of place in the world for individuals living with the condition, however, means that a fuller examination is required. Physical activity can offer the opportunity for individuals to test themselves physically and competitively. Whilst the definition adopted in this article does not prioritise this, it is widely accepted that it can do so. How much individuals living with dementia can achieve for themselves through engaging in physical activity has been found to matter [36]. For example, there are factors such as others having expectations of what individuals might achieve. Such an approach is unlikely to suit everyone; however, people living with dementia report that stereotypical depictions among their peers can lead to their own feelings of stigmatisation [42]. Rather than an overt focus upon goal setting, consideration should be given to other related features found within relevant research. These could include, for example, giving attention to the value that people living with dementia report being invested with and their reports of being noticed through what they did [36]. People living with dementia have also reflected upon the benefits of feeling they "still measured up" ([21], p. 4) through the ability to test this feeling through use of their body. This was found also to involve a sense of mastery over a particular activity, with self-efficacy (the ability to achieve for oneself) being especially prized [21].

However, care needs to be taken when exploring this aspect of the discussion. Throughout, the importance of person-centred approaches has been advanced to run alongside the merits of other features. This is a moment to reflect upon the significance of this because what will suit one person will not be for another. Indeed, a person's preference may vary from one engagement in physical activity to the next [24]. A sense of agency and power can be achieved by people living with dementia participating in physical activity in other ways; for example, as highlighted by Olsen et al. [36], through activity that is challenging but fun. The value individuals report of being able to look forward through ongoing participation over time must also be considered [36]. Conceptualisations of leisure have been applied in such circumstances within the dementia context. For example, "serious leisure" [43] has been used to explain how, through physical activity, individuals have been empowered to acquire and enact skills via the regular progression of activities that are substantial, of interest and fulfilling [44]. If activities feel relevant to the person involved, and if the experiences at the time matter to them, then this may be enough to offer that individual the sense of agency and power required [24].

4. What Should Happen Next?

Physical activity is part of the everyday, particularly with its widely accepted, broadly drawn definition (cited above) to the fore. Thus, it needs to be taken seriously as a means to enable the sustenance of the place in the world of individuals living with dementia. Scholarship from the fields of dementia and physical activity has affirmed this by making the links between physical activity, dementia and the everyday. However, questions remain about the way forward. These relate to matters highlighted in the preceding discussion, but there are also elements that the article has been unable to consider fully enough. In this section, the question of what should happen next is posed. The answers to this and each of the queries raised as part of it will be fundamental to enabling physical activity to realise its fullest potential within the context of life with dementia.

For example, it is not yet clear what skills and attributes are required to offer physical activity to people living with dementia. The articles cited here are helpful in progressing understanding. However, there remains much from the milieu of dementia scholarship and practice that could still contribute. For example, the pioneering work on person-centred practice in dementia [8] has been advanced by others [7] so that person-centred approaches could be understood in theoretical terms and underpin care and support for those living with dementia. In turn, this has enabled good practice to be distilled into resources to enable services and organisations to operationalise what they do (for example, see the "Care Fit for VIPS" framework at https://www.worcester.ac.uk/about/academic-schools/school-of-allied-health-and-community/allied-health-research/association-for-dementia-studies/ads-education-and-research/free-resources/care-fit-for-vips.aspx accessed on 1 February 2023). There is a need for an overarching theory expounding good practice in the facilitation of physical activity for people living with dementia. With initiatives such as social prescribing gaining traction, this would seem timely, especially as the evidence base underpinning it remains uncertain [45].

Who is best placed to be involved in the delivery of physical activity also remains opaque. The authorities drawn upon in this article have not enabled a conclusion to be reached. Some advocated for the involvement of specialists and therapists. For example, Olsen et al. [36] opined that expert knowledge about the aging body is essential. However, as noted above, there is much diversity among people living with dementia, including younger people diagnosed with the condition. The relevance of the aging body would not be so absolute in such instances. Furthermore, might a reliance upon therapy risk the ongoing medicalisation of dementia, a paradigm that has been challenged by established dementia scholarship included within this article [6–8,12]? Better, perhaps, to follow the lead of Burke and Jones [39], who advised that lay people, well briefed, could offer effective opportunities for engagement in physical activity. This could maximise the chance individuals have to participate on an everyday basis, as advocated here. What place within this for family carers? This article has been largely silent on their situation and potential to contribute, focusing the narrative upon the persons themselves. Looking ahead, this is a deficit that requires addressing because, as has been shown, relationships are crucial within the dementia context, and there are no more significant relationships than between those living with dementia and family carers. What role too for people living with dementia themselves in the facilitation of activity? The section exploring collaboration made clear the value of sharing agency and power. More clarity is required about how people themselves can expect to contribute.

Finally, where should physical activity be offered so that people living with dementia gain the most from it? Bearing in mind the preceding discussion, a default answer is likely to be: everywhere feasible within the context of everyday life. That is reasonable and sensible, but places will include hospitals and care/nursing homes. These are venues where people living with dementia spend time, but they are places where control over the physical environment is likely to be limited by constraints, including organisational ones. Leisure and fitness centres, similarly, would seem to offer the opportunity for everyday physical activity. They are under threat from challenges to their resources though [46,47], and work has only just started considering how those spaces can best be used to afford opportunities for good-quality physical activity for people living with dementia [44]. Thus, to answer the question what should happen next, there remains much to consider.

5. Conclusions

This article has highlighted ways in which physical activity can offer more to people living with dementia beyond the physical (important though that is). It has set out ways in which physical activity potentially presents individuals with the wherewithal to sustain their place in the world. To do so, it drew upon scholarship from the dementia field that promotes person-centred approaches to care and support and encouraged consideration of this within the milieu of physical activity. It went further, however. By emphasising the significance of human rights and social citizenship approaches to dementia, the article made the case that physical activity should not be seen as something that is nice and of potential value but as an essential element of everyday life for people living with dementia.

What should happen next is uncertain, as evidenced by the questions posed in the preceding section. What is clear, however, is that physical activity has much to offer to people living with dementia, and at present, its full potential is not being realised. Whether this is because of lack of knowledge, confidence or resources may be uncertain, but the priority must be to consider what is articulated here and use it to enhance the opportunities people living with dementia have to engage in physical activity.

Funding: This research received no external funding.

Institutional Review Board Statement: Not applicable.

Informed Consent Statement: Not applicable.

Data Availability Statement: Data supporting the reported results can be found in the references, which are set out below.

Conflicts of Interest: The author declares no conflict of interest.

References

1. Dening, T.; Sandilyan, M.B. Dementia: Definitions and types. *Nurs. Stand.* **2015**, *29*, 37–42.
2. Alzheimer's Disease International. World Alzheimer Report 2014, Dementia and Risk Reduction. Available online: https://www.alz.co.uk/research/WorldAlzheimerReport2014.pdf (accessed on 12 April 2023).
3. Alzheimer Europe. Behind the headlines: FDA approval of aducanumab marks a watershed moment for the Alzheimer's disease community. *Dement. Eur.* **2021**, *37*, 36–37.
4. New Scientist. Alzheimer's Drug Results are Promising—But not a Major Breakthrough. 2022. Available online: https://www.newscientist.com/article/2340082-alzheimers-drug-results-are-promising-but-not-a-major-breakthrough/ (accessed on 17 April 2023).
5. British Broadcasting Corporation. New Alzheimer's drug Slows Disease by a Third. Available online: https://www.bbc.co.uk/news/health-65471914 (accessed on 3 May 2023).
6. Brooker, D.; Latham, I. *Person-Centred Dementia Care. Making Services Better with the VIPS Framework*, 2nd ed.; Jessica Kingsley Publishers: London, UK, 2016; ISBN 978-1-84905-666-3.
7. Brooker, D. What is person-centred care in dementia? *Rev. Clin. Gerontol.* **2004**, *13*, 215–222. [CrossRef]
8. Kitwood, T. *Dementia Reconsidered. The Person Comes First*; Open University Press: Maidenhead, UK, 1997; ISBN 0335198554.
9. Fletcher, J.R. Destigmatising dementia: The dangers of felt stigma and benevolent othering. *Dementia* **2021**, *20*, 417–426. [CrossRef]
10. Alzheimer's Disease International. World Alzheimer Report 2021, Journey through the Diagnosis of Dementia. p. 19. Available online: https://www.alzint.org/resource/world-alzheimer-report-2021/ (accessed on 12 April 2023).
11. World Health Organization. Global Action Plan on the Public Health Response to Dementia 2017–2025. 2017. Available online: https://www.who.int/publications/i/item/global-action-plan-on-the-public-health-response-to-dementia-2017--2025 (accessed on 12 April 2023).
12. Kitwood, T.; Brooker, D. *Dementia Reconsidered, Revisited; the Person Still Comes First*; Open University Press: London, UK, 2019; ISBN 9780335248025.
13. Fazio, S.; Pace, D.; Flinner, J.; Kalmyer, B. The Fundamentals of Person-Centered Care for Individuals with Dementia. *Gerontologist* **2018**, *58*, S10–S19. [CrossRef]
14. Bartlett, R.; O'Connor, D. From personhood to citizenship: Broadening the lens for dementia practice and research. *J. Aging Stud.* **2007**, *21*, 107–118. [CrossRef]
15. Innovations in Dementia. Our Dementia Our Rights. 2016. Available online: http://www.innovationsindementia.org.uk/wp-content/uploads/2018/01/Our-dementia-Our-rights-booklet.pdf (accessed on 23 April 2023).
16. Bartlett, R.; O'Connor, D. *Broadening the Dementia Debate: Towards Social Citizenship*; Policy Press: London, UK, 2010; ISBN 978-1847421777.
17. Nedlund, C.; Bartlett, R.; Clarke, C. *Everyday Citizenship and People with Dementia*; Dunedin Press: Edinburgh, UK, 2019; ISBN 9781780460826.

18. Bartlett, R.; Brannelly, T. *Life at Home for People with a Dementia*; Routledge: Abingdon, UK, 2019; ISBN 9781138084780.
19. United Nations. Article 30, the Convention on the Rights of Persons with Disabilities. 2008. Available online: https://www.un.org/development/desa/disabilities/convention-on-the-rights-of-persons-with-disabilities/article-30-participation-in-cultural-life-recreation-leisure-and-sport.html (accessed on 29 April 2023).
20. Caspersen, C.J.; Powell, K.E.; Christenson, G.M. Physical activity, exercise, and physical fitness: Definitions and distinctions for health-related research. *Public Health Rep.* **1985**, *100*, 126–131.
21. Clemmensen, T.H.; Lauridsen, H.H.; Andersen-Ranberg, K.; Kristensen, H.K. Informal carers' support needs when caring for a person with dementia–A scoping literature review. *Scand. J. Caring Sci.* **2021**, *35*, 685–700. [CrossRef]
22. Reid, H.; Ridout, A.J.; Tomaz, S.A.; Kelly, P.; Jones, N. Benefits outweigh the risks: A consensus statement on the risks of physical activity for people living with long-term conditions. *Br. J. Sports Med.* **2022**, *56*, 427–438. [CrossRef]
23. Pringle, J.; Jepson, R.; Dawson, A.; McCabe, L.; Bowes, A. How does physical activity benefit people living with dementia? A systematic review to identify the potential mechanisms of action. *Qual. Ageing Older Adults* **2021**, *22*, 3–25. [CrossRef]
24. Tilki, M.; Curran, C.; Burton, L.; Barrett, L. Sport for confidence: A collaborative programme of physical activity, sport and exercise for people with Young Onset Dementia. *Work. Older People* **2022**, *27*, 128–136. [CrossRef]
25. Alty, J.; Farrow, M.; Lawler, K. Exercise and dementia prevention. *Pract. Neurol.* **2020**, *20*, 234–240. [CrossRef]
26. Hartfiel, N.; Gladman, J.; Harwood, R.; Tudor Edwards, R. Social Return on Investment of Home Exercise and Community Referral for People with Early Dementia. *Gerontol. Geriatr. Med.* **2022**, *8*, 1–10. [CrossRef]
27. Shea, S.O. Some Dance to Remember: Exploring the Psychosocial Effects of the Introduction of an Adaptive Irish Céilí Dance Group Activity with People Living with Dementia and their Carers. Master's Dissertation, Technological University of the Shannon Midwest, Limerick, Republic of Ireland, 2021.
28. Rasmussen, J.; Langerman, H. Alzheimer's Disease–Why We Need Early Diagnosis. *Degener. Neurol. Neuromuscul. Dis.* **2019**, *9*, 123–130. [CrossRef]
29. Butchard, S.; Dunne, T.; Engel, H.; Giotsa, A. Stories of human rights Teaching and learning. In *Human Rights Education for Psychologists*, 1st ed.; Hagenaars, P., Plavšić, M., Sveaass, N., Wagner, U., Wainwright, T., Eds.; Routledge: London, UK, 2020; pp. 264–268, ISBN 9780429274312.
30. Cahill, S. *Dementia and Human Rights*; Policy Press: Bristol, UK, 2018; ISBN 9781447331407.
31. Genoe, M.R. Leisure as resistance within the context of Dementia. *Leis. Stud.* **2010**, *29*, 303–320. [CrossRef]
32. Sabat, S. Foreword. In *Dementia and Human Rights*; Cahill, S., Ed.; Policy Press: Bristol, UK, 2018; pp. xi–xiii, ISBN 9781447331407.
33. Barrie, K. Recognition Reconsidered: It is about time. In *Everyday Citizenship and People with Dementia*; Nedlund, C., Bartlett, R., Clarke, C., Eds.; Dunedin Press: Edinburgh, UK, 2019; pp. 13–21, ISBN 9781780460826.
34. Birt, L.; Poland, F.; Csipke, E.; Charlesworth, G. Shifting dementia discourses from deficit to active citizenship. *Sociol. Health Illn.* **2017**, *39*, 199–211. [CrossRef]
35. Kontos, P.; Miller, K.L.; Kontos, A.P. Relational citizenship: Supporting embodied selfhood and relationality in dementia care. *Sociol. Health Illn.* **2017**, *39*, 182–198. [CrossRef]
36. Olsen, C.F.; Telenius, E.W.; Engedal, K.; Bergland, A. Increased self-efficacy: The experience of high-intensity exercise of nursing home residents with dementia—A qualitative study. *BMC Health Serv. Res.* **2015**, *15*, 379. [CrossRef]
37. Telenius, E.W.; Tangen, G.G.; Eriksen, S.; Rokstad, A.M. Fun and a meaningful routine: The experience of physical activity in people with dementia. *BMC Geriatr.* **2022**, *22*, 500. [CrossRef]
38. Wiseman, T. *Leisure in Later Life*; Palgrave Macmillan: Zurich, Switzerland, 2021; ISBN 978-3-030-71671-4.
39. Burke, A.; Jones, A. Pragmatic Evaluation of a Low-Threshold Sports Program for Older Adults in Group Homes. *J. Appl. Gerontol.* **2023**, *42*, 1456–1465. [CrossRef]
40. Elliott, K.-E.J.; Stirling, C.M.; Martin, A.J.; Robinson, A.L.; Scott, J.L. We are not all coping: A cross-sectional investigation of resilience in the dementia care workforce. *Health Expect.* **2016**, *19*, 1251–1264. [CrossRef]
41. Liu, W.; Wang, J. Undergraduate Nursing Students' Willingness of Providing Care for Older Adults with Dementia as Their Future Work. *Innov. Aging* **2021**, *17*, 67. [CrossRef]
42. Dementia Enquirers. Post-Diagnosis Dementia Support: Exploring Experiences and Ideas for Improving Practice. 2022. Available online: https://dementiaenquirers.org.uk/individual-projects/forget-me-not/ (accessed on 29 April 2023).
43. Stebbins, R.A. *Amateurs, Professionals and Serious Leisure*; McGill-Queen's University Press: Montreal, QC, Canada, 1992; ISBN 9780773509016.
44. Russell, C.; Kohe, G.Z.; Evans, S.B.; Brooker, D. Rethinking Spaces of Leisure: How People Living with Dementia Use the Opportunities Leisure Centres Provide to Promote their Identity and Place in the World. *Int. J. Sociol. Leis.* **2022**, *6*, 135–166. [CrossRef]
45. Sandhu, S.; Lian, T.; Connor, D.; Moffatt, S.; Wildman, J.; Wildman, J. Intervention components of link worker social prescribing programmes: A scoping review. *Heath Soc. Care Community* **2022**, *30*, e3761–e3774. [CrossRef]

46. Sport England. Future of Public Sector Leisure. 2022. Available online: https://www.sportengland.org/guidance-and-support/facilities-and-planning/future-public-leisure (accessed on 29 April 2023).
47. UK Active. Leading Bodies for Health, Sport, Fitness and Leisure Urge Prime Minister to Intervene as Grassroots Facilities Face 'Final Straw' If Energy relief Ends. 2023. Available online: https://www.ukactive.com/news/leading-bodies-for-health-sport-fitness-and-leisure-urge-prime-minister-to-intervene-as-grassroots-facilities-face-final-straw-if-energy-relief-ends/ (accessed on 29 April 2023).

Disclaimer/Publisher's Note: The statements, opinions and data contained in all publications are solely those of the individual author(s) and contributor(s) and not of MDPI and/or the editor(s). MDPI and/or the editor(s) disclaim responsibility for any injury to people or property resulting from any ideas, methods, instructions or products referred to in the content.

MDPI AG
Grosspeteranlage 5
4052 Basel
Switzerland
Tel.: +41 61 683 77 34

International Journal of Environmental Research and Public Health Editorial Office
E-mail: ijerph@mdpi.com
www.mdpi.com/journal/ijerph

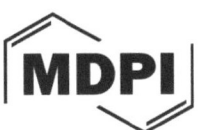

Disclaimer/Publisher's Note: The title and front matter of this reprint are at the discretion of the Guest Editors. The publisher is not responsible for their content or any associated concerns. The statements, opinions and data contained in all individual articles are solely those of the individual Editors and contributors and not of MDPI. MDPI disclaims responsibility for any injury to people or property resulting from any ideas, methods, instructions or products referred to in the content.

www.ingramcontent.com/pod-product-compliance
Lightning Source LLC
LaVergne TN
LVHW072359090526
838202LV00019B/2582